THE DOSE MAKES THE POISON

The
DOSE
makes the
POISON

A Plain-Language Guide
to Toxicology

Second Edition

M. Alice Ottoboni, Ph.D.

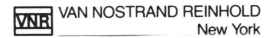 VAN NOSTRAND REINHOLD
New York

Van Nostrand Reinhold
115 Fifth Avenue
New York, New York 10003

Chapman and Hall
2-6 Boundary Row
London, SE1 8HN, England

Thomas Nelson Australia
102 Dodds Street
South Melbourne 3205
Victoria, Australia

Nelson Canada
1120 Birchmount Road
Scarborough, Ontario MIK 5G4, Canada

16 15 14 13 12 11 10 9 8 7 6 5 4 3

Library of Congress Cataloging-in-Publication Data

Ottoboni, M. Alice.
    The dose makes the poison: a plain-language guide to toxicology/
  M. Alice Ottoboni.—2nd ed.
        p. cm.

    Includes bibliographical references and index.
    ISBN 0-442-00660-8
    1. Toxicology—Popular works. I. Title.
    [DNLM: 1. Toxicology—popular works. QV 600 091d]
  RA1213.088 1991
  615.9—dc20
  DNLM/DLC
  for Library of Congress   91-7239
                                                               CIP

CONTENTS

10/10

10/17

PREFACE

When the first edition of this book was published in 1984, I thought that the public's fear of environmental chemicals had peaked. It seemed that the need for a book explaining toxicology in lay terms had passed and that such a book would no longer be of value. Time has proved me wrong; poison paranoia has continued to grow and flourish. The general public seems more concerned than ever about environmental chemicals.

The public's fear of chemicals, combined with increasing government and industry recognition that people must be protected from harmful exposures to chemicals, has resulted in a dramatic increase during the past decade in the number of laws regulating environmental chemicals. The majority of these laws were written by legislators and other public officials who recognized the need for regulation of chemicals and who also understood that sound planning and management were essential in the design of legislation to protect environmental and public health. Laws enacted by legislatures are subjected to extensive review and refinement prior to passage. During the review process, legislators receive the benefit of scientific input and public comment.

A few of the laws regulating chemicals that have been passed in recent years were not the result of the legislative process. They were enacted through the initiative process, a procedure by which the public is able to enact legislation at the ballot box. Initiatives are written by a sponsoring group and submitted to the public in petition form. They are placed on the ballot if their petitions receive the required number of signatures. Initiatives are subject only to political debate. They do not receive the benefits of public legislative hearings and review. If they become law, they are fairly well protected from legislative modification.

In states that have the initiative process, organizations who consider that governmental officials are indifferent to environmental pollution have bypassed the legislative process and have gone directly to the people with initiatives to regulate more stringently or eliminate the use of chemicals, particularly chemicals used as pesticides. These campaigns have benefited by exploiting the public's fear of chemicals. The success of the initiative process demonstrates that fear and emotion can be very effective in stimulating public action. The ability of environmental laws based on fear and emotion, rather than reason and knowledge, to deliver what they promise, namely increased public and environmental health protection, has yet to be demonstrated. In fact, they may well be antiproductive because they divert resources and energies away from sound environmental legislation and policies. The prudence and wisdom of centuries tell us that lasting and viable solutions to any societal problem can only come from reason and knowledge.

The initiative process makes the need for an informed public more critical than ever. Initiatives require citizens to make extremely important decisions that will affect their lives and those of future generations. Sound decisions require an understanding and knowledge of all sides of issues.

This book was written in the belief that knowledge of what makes chemicals harmful can help dispel unreasoning fear and can aid in dealing more effectively with real problems. I have found, from my many years of working for and with the public, that most people are intelligent and perceptive individuals who want scientific facts relating to subjects that are vital to their health and well-being. Even without scientific education, they are completely capable of understanding such facts. This book is for them. Its purpose is to provide facts about the toxicity of chemicals to help people cope with news media toxicology, preserve their sanity in the face of poison paranoia, and make informed judgments about chemicals in the environment.

The second edition contains essentially all of the information presented in the first edition, but, hopefully, in a more organized manner. For example, all of the experimental and analytical methods mentioned in several chapters in the first edition are collected in Chapter 12. References to the origins of toxicology and regulation of chemicals are brought together in Chapter 3. In addition to reorganization, subjects such as public distrust of science, epidemiology, and risk have been expanded because they are subjects of increasing importance to an understanding of toxicology and its relationship to current environmental problems.

As with the first edition, the information presented in this book is based on common toxicological knowledge; thus, it does not contain many references. References are given in those instances where other authors, publications, or specific studies are mentioned. In addition, a Suggested Reading section is provided at the end of the book for people who wish to pursue particular topics.

Again, I must explain to feminist readers who may object to the use of the masculine gender throughout the book that I had difficulty in dealing with this issue. The use of terms like he/she, man/woman, his/hers, and so forth makes for very cumbersome reading without enhancing the clarity of any point. In the absence of nouns and pronouns that carry no sex identification (with the exception of human, person, and the plural pronouns, all of which are used liberally throughout the book) I decided to use masculine forms and explain that I intend them in a generic sense.

I am grateful to the many friends and associates with whom I have discussed this second edition for their very valuable comments and criticisms. I owe a special debt of gratitude to my husband Fred. His sharing of his knowledge of public, occupational, and environmental health has been of tremendous benefit to me not only in the preparation of this second edition but in all of my professional activities.

INTRODUCTION

Many years of service as a public health toxicologist for the California Department of Public Health (now the Department of Health Services) made it disturbingly clear to me that an inordinate fear of chemicals was the rule rather than the exception among the general public. During the same years, participation in training programs designed to teach people how to work safely with the chemicals they contacted in their occupations taught me that people with no science background were not only capable of understanding the basic principles of toxicology but that they could also apply what they learned to work safely and comfortably with some very dangerous chemicals. This book was born of these two observations.

There is a general lack of public understanding about what makes chemicals toxic, and about the word that has become a synonym for *toxic*. That word, now a part of our everyday vocabulary, is *poison*. Headlines tell us about the poisons in our food, poisons in our water, poisons in our air—poisons everywhere! People who use the word most freely appear to have the least concept of what poison means. The indiscriminate use of the word has brought us into an era of what might be termed poison paranoia.

Whenever some misfortune occurs for which we have no ready explanation—an illness, a mischance of nature, a declining wildlife species—we look to blame some chemical. This propensity is aptly illustrated by the mystery of the double-yolked eggs, reported in the Consumers Cooperative of Berkeley newspaper, the *Co-op News*, July 16, 1979: "Science is beautiful, but it can sometimes spoil a good news story." The story went on to tell that a Co-op member

> . . . was recently amazed when she found NINE double eggs out of a dozen box. I shared her astonishment, convinced that either

1

the odds against this marvelous happening were billions to one or that some horrible chemical additive fed to a chicken had caused it, and that some serious muckraking was needed down at the chicken ranch to protect embattled consumers by eliminating this poison from their diet.

The Co-op home economist checked with the supplier of the eggs and received a reply

. . . that took all of the mystery out of the event by placing it squarely in the dull world of young chickens and egg sorting, where neither chemicals nor miraculous odds were at issue.

Young chickens are apt to pop more eggs with two yolks, but it becomes more uncommon as they reach maturity. The reason nine eggs could wind up in the same box is because double eggs are oversized, so they get set aside by the egg sorter because they won't fit in the egg container. However, there are some borderline ones which the sorter selects from those set aside and allows to pass through. This is why so many were in one box.

Fortunately, in the case of the double-yolked eggs, further facts were sought and the real reason for the apparent anomaly was discovered, thereby avoiding another scare headline. Unfortunately, such dedication in pursuit of truth is often the exception rather than the rule.

There are two diametrically opposed dangers in news media toxicology and its offspring, poison paranoia. One is the cry-wolf syndrome. When an alarm is sounded frequently and without regard to degree of emergency, the alarm becomes meaningless and, therefore, is not effective when a true emergency exists. It is well known that to call everything bad, in effect, is to call nothing bad. If safe and sane use of chemicals in our homes, work, and recreation places is to be furthered, there must be understanding, cooperation, and support on the part of the public. A public blasé about harmful effects of chemicals is a public disinterested in making any changes in use practices relating to chemicals. Such a public attitude would be tragic.

The second danger is that a certain fraction of our population will become victims of a helpless, hopeless fear and terror that chemicals from which they cannot escape—chemicals in their food, their water, their air—are destroying their health, shortening their lives, or dooming them to cancer. Such a fear is a form of stress that can be just as damaging as the chemicals that are feared, and in some cases even more so. Stress can produce vague feelings of illness, such as nausea, headache, weakness, and malaise, as well as actual physical illness. The medical profession now generally accepts the premise that stress can exert a profound influence on the course of many illnesses. Stress can actually be an etiologic (causative) agent for some cases of such diseases as high blood pressure, ulcers, allergies, colitis, and even cancer.

Poison paranoia already is taking a toll in the mental health and well-being of some people. This conclusion is based on the many thousands of calls, letters, and visits that I have received from people concerned about the health effects of chemicals in their environments. The gamut of their concern extended from calm interest to outright panic. In a few cases, the cause for apprehension was valid because, through some accident, misuse, or lack of knowledge, there had been an actual or potential exposure to a harmful level of some chemical. However, in the majority of cases, the fears or concerns were ill-defined and prompted, in the main, by the most recent scare headline. Among the latter, there were a few people who refused to accept any information that did not support their conviction that they were suffering from some sort of chemical poisoning. People who fall victim to an unreasonable fear of chemicals are literally frightened sick. Frightened people truly suffer. They are victims of distorted information and lack of knowledge.

The great majority of people are seriously concerned about the many chemicals reported to be harming them and the environment, but they do not have a pathologic fear about the effects of chemicals on their health. For the most part, they do not know what to do about the situation, other than to modify their life-styles to the extent possible. They can live without smoking, but they cannot live without breathing.

This book is not intended as a condemnation of, or an apology for, synthetic chemicals; rather its aim is to present an objective discussion of what makes chemicals harmful or harmless. I feel compelled to make this point so that the reader will understand that I hold no brief for or against synthetic chemicals; they are facts of life with which we must deal. I have learned from many years of contact with people of all viewpoints regarding the risks posed by chemicals that objectivity often invites scorn from both extremes of view. Thus, both pro- and antichemical extremists may take exception to all or parts of this book because it is not directed toward reinforcement of their respective "what's-the-fuss" and "ain't-it-awful" views. This book is not written for people of extreme persuasions, but rather for people who want a real understanding of the significance of their many chemical exposures. Only people with open minds are tolerant of concepts that are new to them or in conflict with their beliefs.

The comfort provided by knowledge was vividly brought home to me many years ago by a young woman who called for information about a chemical. After a rather lengthy conversation, she said, "I feel so sorry for you. You know so much about all the harmful effects of the chemicals that surround us that you must really worry all the time."

I was surprised by her statement, because such a thought had never occurred to me. I assured her that, on the contrary, the very fact that I do know what makes chemicals harmful frees me from worry. All chemicals follow the same rules—the laws of nature. By knowing the rules, I have a perspective that protects me from needless worry and unreasoning fear. My hope is that this book will give you the same perspective.

1

WHAT ARE CHEMICALS?

The word *chemical* has become a dirty word in our modern American vocabulary. Our public media provide us daily with advice or warnings about the presence of chemicals in our food, air, and water, and the harm they are doing to us and the world we live in. As a result, the word *chemical* conjures up visions of damage, debility, disease, and death in the minds of many people. In order to truly understand the threats posed by chemicals—a prerequisite to dealing wisely in protecting ourselves and our environment from adverse effects of chemicals—we must clarify or reform our concept of the word *chemical*.

ATOMS AND MOLECULES

All matter is composed of chemical elements. An individual unit of an element is called an atom. Atoms are the basic building blocks for all substances. There are approximately 90 different kinds of stable elements found in nature. Examples of elements are hydrogen, oxygen, carbon, nitrogen, gold, and silver. A complete listing of all of the elements, including those that are unstable (radioactive), can be found in any good dictionary. A multicolored diagram of the periodic table of elements that explains how the periodic table is constructed and the relationships among the elements appeared in the December 1989 issue of *National Geographic* (176(6):757–759).

When two or more atoms (usually of different elements) are linked together by chemical bonding, they form units called molecules. A substance composed of molecules all of the same kind is called a compound. Water, salt, and sugar are examples of compounds. The number of different kinds of molecules that can be formed by the combination of from 2 to many thousands of atoms, from more than 90 different elements, is astronomical. All substances are composed of chemical and physical combinations of atoms (elements) and molecules (compounds). Thus, everything in our physical world is chemical—the food we eat, the water we drink, the clothes we wear, the medicines we take, the cosmetics we use, the plants in our garden, our furniture, our homes, our automobiles, and even ourselves. Our entire physical world is composed of chemicals.

SYNTHETIC CHEMICALS

Once we accept the fact that all things are chemical, we come to the realization that what people really are concerned about are not chemicals, but man-made chemicals. Humans, in their ingenuity, have been able to take the basic building blocks of which all matter is composed and link them together in new combinations to produce compounds not found in nature. Thus, we have a host of synthetic substances, primarily organic, available to us, which we put to a seemingly endless variety of uses—pharmaceuticals, pesticides, and polymers of all sorts, including the common household plastics with which we are so familiar, to name just a few.

The term *organic* has been extensively misused by the health-food industry and, as a result, is generally misunderstood by the public. Organic has come to mean something (usually food) that is naturally occurring or produced without the use of pesticides or other synthetic chemicals. In reality, organic chemicals are simply chemicals composed primarily of the element carbon, independent of whether they are natural or synthetic. It comes as a shock to many people that almost all synthetic chemicals, including pesticides, are organic chemicals.

The term *organic* was coined long before the birth of modern chemistry. Early scientists who studied the composition of matter recognized that substances produced by living organisms were different from all other chemicals then known to man. They called the former organic (derived from organisms) as opposed to the latter, which they classed as inorganic. Early in the nineteenth century, it was discovered that the element carbon was present in all organic compounds; hence carbon chemistry became synonymous with organic chemistry.

The great complexity of carbon chemistry, relative to inorganic chemistry, the large size and complicated structures of many organic compounds, their great number and variety, combined with the fact that organic chemicals were only found in living organisms or products of living organisms, led the early-day chemists to endow organic chemicals with mystical properties. They considered that the laws that governed the behavior of inorganic chemicals did not apply to organic chemicals; humans could synthesize inorganic compounds, but were incapable of synthesizing organic compounds in the laboratory.

The special properties of organic chemicals were attributed to the action of a supernatural force, the "vital force," as distinct from the crude and vulgar forces that governed inorganic chemicals. Berzelius, a noted chemist of the early nineteenth century, wrote that the vital force was unrelated to inorganic elements and determined none of their characteristic properties. Berzelius considered that the vital force was a mysterious property beyond comprehension.

The birth of synthetic organic chemistry occurred at about the time of Berzelius' writing, with the first laboratory synthesis of an organic chemical, using inorganic chemicals as starting materials. The first synthetic organic chemical was oxalic acid, made by the German chemist Friedrich Wöhler. A short time later, Wöhler also synthesized urea. After this accomplishment, Wöhler wrote to Berzelius to tell him that he had prepared urea, a chemical found in the urine of animals "without requiring a kidney or animal, either man or dog."

The notion that organic and inorganic chemicals were qualitatively different persisted for decades after the revolutionary demonstration that humans could, indeed, synthesize organic chemicals. The science of chemistry was greatly retarded until the chemical properties of carbon and its place in the periodic table were more fully understood.

The great numbers of synthetic organic chemicals that have been created since the end of World War II have not been of much public interest until recent years. The publication of Rachel Carson's book *Silent Spring* (Boston: Houghton Mifflin), in 1962, stimulated great interest in the effects of pesticides on environmental and public health, and brought to public attention what is now known as a proliferation of chemicals.

The number and variety of synthetic organic chemicals are truly amazing. In 1978 there were over four million organic and inorganic chemicals listed in the American Chemical Society's registry of chemicals. More than 95 percent of these chemicals are organic. Of all the known organic chemicals, perhaps half are naturally occurring chemicals that have been synthesized in the laboratory or isolated from natural sources. An article in the June 1983 issue of *Popular Science* (p. 11) mentioned that the six-millionth chemical produced since 1965 had just been recorded.

For the average person, what is the significance of the existence of more than six million chemicals? Among those that are not naturally occurring, the great majority are what might be considered chemical oddities; they exist only in small quantities in vials on chemists' benches or in chemical storerooms. They have not been found to have any practical use or function and so have never been developed commercially.

The toxicity of synthetic chemicals covers the entire range of toxicity from essentially nontoxic to extremely toxic. Some synthetic chemicals, such as artificial sweeteners, are edible, whereas others, such as chemical warfare agents, are lethal in extremely small amounts. Regardless of degree of toxicity, the principles of toxicology apply equally to all chemicals, whether synthetic or natural.

The number of chemicals that actually enter homes is not known, but a survey of the wide variety of products found in the home setting—such as cleansers, polishes, drugs, cosmetics, prepared foods, pesticides and other garden chemicals, automotive products, and hobby products—would indicate that the number is quite large. Despite the wide variety of products, many contain the same basic chemicals. Thus, the actual number of individual chemicals that the average person comes in contact with in home products is probably much closer to several thousand than several million. The majority of chemicals that are permitted to enter homes are not harmful when used properly, but some are treated with a more cavalier attitude than is warranted, as witnessed by the numerous accidental poisonings that occur in children.

The people who contact the widest variety of potentially dangerous chemicals are the people in businesses or professions that use chemicals in some process or procedure and the people who work in industries that synthesize, manufacture, formulate, or use chemicals to make other products. Few of these chemicals find their way into a home setting.

NATURAL CHEMICALS

The total number of chemical compounds in our universe that occur naturally will probably never be known exactly, but, from the millions that have been identified thus far, we know that the total number must be almost unimaginable. Natural chemicals may be organic or inorganic. Our inanimate world is an inorganic world. It is composed of a great number of mineral substances in which all of the elements, except for a few radioactive elements that have been created by nuclear scientists, are represented.

Our living world is composed primarily of organic compounds, the diversity of which is tremendously greater than that in our inorganic world. The number of natural organic compounds that has been identified thus far, although very large, is probably negligible compared to the number of those yet unidentified. Many of these as-yet unidentified organic chemicals, components of the trees, shrubs, and other plants of the rain forests, could well be of great value to medical and pharmaceutical sciences.

One small segment of our organic world, food plants and animals, provide us with the nutrients that we use to build and repair our bodies. However, the plants and animals we use for food contain many more natural chemicals than just the nutrients we require. Since it is impossible to separate nutrients from nonnutrients in our foods, we depend on our bodies to do this work for us. There are many kinds and quantities of nonnutrients in our foods, particularly our plant foods. The animals we use for food have already done the job for us of selecting nutrients and eliminating most of the nonnutrients from plants.

Among the natural chemicals that we eat there are many that can cause adverse effects if consumed in excess. In fact, there is probably no food that does not contain some potentially harmful natural chemical. This fact is the basis for an annual project of the American Council on Science and Health. Every fall they publish a typical Thanksgiving menu accompanied by identification of the naturally occurring toxic or carcinogenic chemicals present in each food on the menu.

An interesting method for ranking the potential health effects from exposure to toxicants that occur naturally in foods has been developed by Bruce Ames and his colleagues at the University of California, Berkeley. Dr. Ames has written numerous articles for both scientific and popular publications reviewing the subject of naturally occurring toxicants and their carcinogenic hazards. Rankings are based on data from the scientific literature, as well as from Dr. Ames' own laboratory, using accepted methods of risk assessment. These rankings are one approach to the evaluation of relative health risks posed by suspected carcinogens, both natural and synthetic.

CHEMICAL CATEGORIES

We categorize chemicals in many different ways, the broadest of which is whether they are natural, produced by a living process, or synthetic, made by humans. Other ways we classify chemicals are by the use we make of them (foods, drugs, pesticides, etc.), how they are physically organized (solid, liquid, gas), what kind of animal they are (fish, reptiles, birds, mammals, etc.), whether they are organic or inorganic (animal, vegetable, or mineral), and so forth. Plant and animal probably were two of the earliest categories recognized by humans. Plants stayed put, whereas animals moved about freely.

A scheme of classification by the use we make of a chemical or product is essential for government regulation of such items as foods, drugs, cosmetics, pesticides, industrial chemicals, and medical devices. If a substance is claimed to be a food, it is governed by the food laws. If the exact same substance is packaged and labeled a drug, it is governed by the drug laws, not by the food laws; the laws that pertain depend on what use the manufacturer or seller specifies for the product. For example, hydrochloric acid is regulated as a household product when it is present in cleaning compounds, as a drug when it is used to treat people with low gastric acidity, as a hazardous industrial chemical when it is used in electroplating, and as a pesticide adjuvant when it is used to enhance the germicidal activity of chlorine in swimming pools. Hydrochloric acid is natural when produced by the stomach and synthetic when made in the laboratory.

Another example is boric acid, which occurs naturally as the mineral sassolite, but also can be synthesized in the laboratory. It is regulated as a household product when used in laundry detergents, as a drug when sold as an antiseptic eyewash, as an insecticide when used to kill roaches, as an herbicide when applied to kill weeds, and as a flame retardant when used to fireproof fabrics. Many chemicals, like hydrochloric acid and boric acid, fall into both drug and pesticide categories. Coumarin compounds, such as warfarin, are not only excellent rodenticides but are also valuable anticoagulant drugs that are used to prevent blood clots. DDD, a close relative of DDT—the infamous pesticide now banned in the United States—and itself an insecticide, has been used therapeutically to treat certain forms of adrenal cancer.

Hopefully, the important lesson to be learned from these examples is apparent: The physical, chemical, and toxicologic properties of any chemical are totally independent of the category in which it is placed. The toxicity of boric acid is exactly the same when it is used as a drug as it is when it is used as a pesticide.

PESTICIDES—A SPECIAL CATEGORY

Although some people are concerned about the products and effluents from the chemical industry, the class of man-made chemicals that is almost universally dreaded is the category known as pesticides. Pesticides are substances, natural or synthetic, that are used to kill some pest—a plant, animal, insect, or other organism that has been determined to be undesirable for some economic, medical, or esthetic reason. Included in the pesticide category are insecticides, fungicides, herbicides, rodenticides, germicides, and a whole host of other "-cides."

There are countless chemicals that are as toxic, or more so, than many of the pesticides, but the focus of fear centers on this group. Why? One probable reason is the tremendous amount of publicity given to reports of damage from the presence of pesticides in our environment and even in our own bodies. Another probable reason is that pesticides are used to kill living things, and thus are labeled as poisons in the public mind. The concept of poison is considered by many people to be an all-or-none phenomenon; a chemical is either a poison or it is not, with no shades of gray in between. Nothing could be further from the truth. Such simplistic reasoning is counterproductive to an understanding of how and why chemicals cause harm. It also points up the fallacy of assigning blanket judgments of safety or harm to categories of chemicals.

CHEMICALS—"GOOD" AND "BAD"

A common misconception that must be overcome before an understanding of toxicity can be achieved is that chemicals made by nature are good and those made by man are bad. Actually, toxicologists recognize that Mother Nature is far more ingenious than man could ever be in devising toxic chemicals. She is not only far more ingenious but she is also much more prolific; of all the chemicals that exist, the number that are natural far exceeds the number made by humans. In addition, there are tens to hundreds of thousands of plants that botanists have not even identified yet, much less characterized chemically. The voluminous literature on the toxic properties of naturally occurring chemicals that have been identified in food and nonfood plants, animals, and microorganisms supports an estimate that the fraction of natural chemicals that are toxic is at least as great as the fraction of synthetic chemicals that are toxic.

Some of the most toxic chemicals that exist are produced by living organisms. A good example is botulin, the toxin produced by *Clostridium botulinum* organisms. One milligram (mg) of botulin ($\frac{1}{28}$ thousandth of an ounce) is capable of killing 20 million mice. It is estimated that the average lethal dose of botulin for an adult human is 2 micrograms (μg), or $\frac{1}{14}$ millionth of an ounce, a very, very tiny amount.

Toxic chemicals of natural origin, such as those produced by algae and other microorganisms, snakes and other venomous animals, and plants, constitute a more common threat to wild and domestic species than do man-made chemicals. Actually, natural and synthetic chemicals together are probably far less detrimental to wildlife species than habitat destruction resulting from encroachment by civilization and the burgeoning human populations.

Although man-made chemicals form a far smaller group than natural chemicals, they have become the symbols for the damage that the human species is inflicting on the planet Earth and all its inhabitants. Why have synthetic chemicals, as apart from natural chemicals, been singled out for this distinction? One reason may be that humans have been irresponsible, often unknowingly, in their use and disposal of synthetic chemicals, the relatively new products and tools of their civilization. As a result, problems of air, water, and general environmental pollution have been visited on societies throughout the world. Further, because synthetic chemicals are created by humans, there is a sense that they can be controlled by humans. The synthesis of new chemicals can be prevented and the production of old chemicals can be halted.

A second reason may relate to the general feeling that natural chemicals pose no threat. The theory is that man and animals evolved with natural chemicals and are therefore adapted to them. This theory is not in accord with known adverse effects of natural chemicals in humans, such as the carcinogenicity of certain mold toxins or the acute toxicity of chemicals produced by a variety of microorganisms.

WHY THE "GOOD–BAD" DICHOTOMY?

What are the properties of synthetic chemicals that have fostered the dichotomy of man-made (bad) versus natural (good)? An exploration of this question is important to an understanding of the effects of chemicals on living organisms.

The attributes of synthetic chemicals that set them apart from chemicals of natural origin were elegantly described over a decade ago by Barry Commoner:

> The clash between the economic success of synthetic petrochemicals and their increasing vulnerability to biological complaints is the inevitable result of the fact that they are synthetic—made by man, not nature. In every living cell there is a tightly integrated network of chemical processes which has evolved over three billion years of trial and error. In all of the countless organisms that have ever lived over this time, and in all of their even more numerous cells, there has been a huge number of opportunities for chemical errors—the production of substances that could disrupt the delicately balanced chemistry of the living cell. Like other evolutionary misfits, any organism that made these chemical mistakes perished, so that the genetic tendency to produce the offending substance was eliminated from the line of evolutionary descent. One can imagine that at some point in the course of evolution some unfortunate cell managed to synthesize, let us say DDT—and became a casualty in the evolutionary struggle to survive.
>
> Another requirement for evolutionary survival is that every substance synthesized by living things must be broken down by them as well—be biodegradable. It is this rule which establishes the dis-

tinctive closed cycles of ecology. When petrochemical technology synthesizes a new complex substance that is alien to living things, they are likely to lack the enzymes needed to degrade the substance—which then accumulates as waste. This explains why our beaches have become blanketed in debris, since nondegradable synthetics have replaced hemp, cordage, wooden spoons and paper cups, which, because they were made of natural cellulose, soon decayed.

The likelihood that a synthetic organic chemical will be biologically hazardous increases with its complexity; the more elaborate its structure, the more likely that some part of it will be incompatible with the normal chemistry of life. (The promise and perils of petrochemicals, *New York Times Magazine,* September 25, 1977, p. 38)

We can distill from this essay three attributes that make man-made chemicals biologically undesirable: They are made by man, not nature, they are not biodegradable, and they tend to be of very complex structure. None of these attributes bear any relationship to toxicity or the ability of a chemical to do harm. Let us examine each individually to explain why.

Man-Made Chemicals Are Man-Made

The first attribute, man-made chemicals are harmful because they are man-made, is a commonly held opinion. It is an example of a form of reasoning that, in logic, is known as *circulus in probando,* or, literally, "a circle in the proof." Water is wet because it is water, man is human because he is man, and truth is good because it is truth are examples of circular reasoning. Such logic adds nothing to the argument that synthetic chemicals are biologically damaging. It returns us to the dichotomy of man-made (bad) versus natural (good) without adding anything to our knowledge of why the dichotomy exists or of its validity.

The hypothetical cell described above as perishing in some eon past because it committed the blunder of synthesizing DDT, a complex man-made organic compound with insecticidal properties, is worthy of a moment's reflection. This unfortunate cell is intended to serve as a dramatic, and perhaps whimsical, example of the undesirability of synthetic chemicals. However, the lamentable cell could never be more than a creature of fiction because its tale is founded in fancy rather than fact. The reality is that living cells do not just suddenly synthesize highly complex molecules. Complex natural molecules are the end product of many biochemical reactions occurring in well-coordinated sequence.

The building of a complex molecule by a living organism may be likened to the building of an automobile on an assembly line. At each step along the way, some small change or addition is made until, finally, at the end of the line, an automobile emerges. So it is with complex biochemicals: Each reaction in a biochemical chain makes some small change or addition to the molecule produced by the preceding reaction. This process is repeated numerous times, with each reaction producing the precursor for the next reaction in the chain, until, finally, a complex biochemical molecule is synthesized.

If all intermediary precursor biochemicals are compatible with cellular life, it is highly unlikely that the final step in the synthesis would produce a biochemical lethal to the cell. Thus, if the hypothetical cell described above did manage to synthesize DDT, it probably would be unaffected by the presence of DDT within itself. If the unfortunate cell were a plant cell, its destiny might be radically changed. Consider the tremendous survival advantage that a built-in insecticide would confer on a plant! The idea of a plant cell producing an insecticidal chemical is not as absurd as it may seem on the surface; pyrethrins and nicotine, produced by chrysanthemums and tobacco, respectively, are commercially available insecticides.

The concept that chemicals are good or bad depending on their origin (nature or the laboratory) requires that chemicals possess an inherent moral quality of "goodness" or "badness," which, of course, is absurd. Morality is a creation of the human mind and applies only to human conduct—not to inanimate things such as chemicals. The anthropomorphic view that nature, evolution, living cells, or inanimate objects are endowed with human sensibilities is out of context with reality. Such a view of cellular functions or natural processes is common among primitive cultures and medicine men. Scientists may use the term *Mother Nature,* or credit natural processes with intelligence, as a figure of speech for literary effect, but they do not invoke the gods to explain phenomena outside their areas of scientific expertise.

The distinction between natural and man-made chemicals is actually a man-made distinction. Living cells are not conscious units capable of deciding whether molecules that enter them are natural or synthetic. Our bodies cannot recognize the origin of a chemical—Mother Nature or the chemical laboratory. Our bodies can only distinguish between molecules they can use (for energy or to make more of themselves, more muscle, more bone, more blood, etc.) and molecules they cannot use. The former we call biochemicals and the latter we call foreign, or xenobiotic, chemicals.

Biochemicals may be natural or man-made, and foreign chemicals may be natural or man-made. The distinction between biochemicals and foreign chemicals exists for all living organisms, and varies among classes of organisms. What may be a biochemical for one class of living things may be a foreign chemical for others. For example, strychnine is a natural chemical produced by nux vomica plants. Thus it is a biochemical for nux vomica plants, but a foreign chemical (and a deadly one at that) for animal species, including humans. Although strychnine is a very toxic chemical for many species for which it is foreign, foreign chemicals are not of necessity harmful. The toxicity of chemicals does not correlate with their origin—nature or the chemical laboratory. Both natural and synthetic chemicals have wide ranges of toxicity, with large areas of overlap.

Man-Made Chemicals Are Not Biodegradable

The second attribute of man-made chemicals that allegedly makes them undesirable is their lack of biodegradability. Biodegradation refers to the process by which living organisms break down (metabolize) complex molecules to simpler molecules. In actual fact, there are relatively few man-made compounds that are not metabolized to some degree by some living organisms. All higher animals, including humans, have very complex sets of enzyme systems that process xenobiotic chemicals. Among the synthetic compounds that are most resistant to biodegradation are the long-chain polymers that we know as plastics. As a class, the plastics are nontoxic. Some are sufficiently inert biologically to be implanted surgically as substitutes for blood vessels, bone, and other living structures.

Like synthetic polymers, there are some substances produced by natural processes that are equally resistant to biodegradation, such as the skeletons of diatoms, sea shells, bones, and hair. Thus, the bones of prehistoric man and animals can be studied by archeologists today, thousands and thousands of years after their owners walked upon the Earth. And Napoleon's hair was still intact 140 years after his death, to be available to chemists for arsenic analysis to test the theory that Napoleon died of arsenic poisoning.

Chemicals, both natural and synthetic, that are resistant to biodegradation may be either toxic or nontoxic. If they are toxic, they enter the organism and do damage because they are not converted to a less toxic form. If they are nontoxic, they enter and do no damage because they are not converted to a more toxic form. In both cases, they are essentially unchanged by their passage through the organism. Chemicals, both natural and synthetic, that are biodegradable may also be either toxic or nontoxic. Some that are themselves nontoxic may be converted into toxic compounds during the process of metabolism. For these chemicals, biodegradability is a disadvantage to an organism; the process of biodegradation produces toxins. Other chemicals that are themselves toxic may be metabolically converted to less toxic or nontoxic compounds. For these chemicals, biodegradability is an advantage, and the process is called detoxification. Biodegradability and toxicity are independent properties of chemicals.

Nonbiodegradable junk may offend our esthetic senses when it "blankets our beaches in debris,'' but plastic spoons and cups are no more esthetically offensive than wooden spoons and paper cups which, if not picked up and discarded, seem to have as long a residence time as junk as do their plastic counterparts. The plastic counterparts may soon become more quickly degradable than paper or wood if industry's successes in making biodegradable plastics become a practical reality.

Most foreign objects, whether they are made of natural or synthetic materials, have the potential to harm any creature that ingests, inhales, or becomes entangled in them. The damage that has been done to some marine birds and mammals by plastic articles relates primarily to their form or shape. Children who play with thin plastic bags are also at risk if they put the bags over their heads and faces. They may suffocate because the plastic film does not permit air exchange. Plastics are themselves nontoxic, but they can cause physical damage.

Biodegradable plastics may not solve the ecological problem completely. A seal pup with its mouth held shut by a six-pack ring cannot wait a few weeks or even a few months for the ring to decompose. Changes in design of containers and packaging may be required as well as changes in the composition of the materials used. However, the problem of plastic litter is as much a societal problem as an industry one. We must accept the responsibility for proper disposal of debris that may harm some creature. It does not take much time to cut open six-pack rings or tie knots in plastic bags.

Further, the damage done by plastic debris to fish, fowl, and aquatic organisms, as well as to the esthetic beauty of our beaches, is small compared to that done by crude oil spilled from tankers, accidentally or deliberately, or released during blowouts from offshore wells. Crude oil, a raw material for synthetic chemicals, is not man-made, but produced by natural processes from once-living organisms. Some components of crude oil, all of which are natural, are notably resistant to biodegradation, as any resident of a coastal town plagued by an oil spill will attest. An example of a useful crude oil derivative that is resistant to biodegradation is asphalt, which is used to pave our streets.

A property of chemicals that results from a lack of biodegradability is persistence, the ability to remain in the environment unchanged by such factors as light, temperature, or microorganisms. Environmental concerns about persistence are related almost entirely to pesticides that are persistent. It is a desirable quality in pesticides, from the viewpoint of effectiveness and efficiency. A pesticide that retains its ability to kill pests for prolonged periods need be applied less often than one that degrades rapidly. Thus, the total quantity of pesticide required to do a job is considerably less, which reduces the cost of crop protection and production.

The undesirable aspects of persistence in pesticides relate to their continued pesticidal action after such need ceases to exist, and to the fact that they remain in the environment for prolonged periods. The majority of persistent chlorinated hydrocarbon pesticides, such as DDT, have been banned from use in the United States because they were considered responsible for declines in the populations of certain wildlife species.

The rationale that substitution of nonpersistent pesticides for persistent ones will solve all of the environmental problems attributed to the latter is an example of the myopic thinking that permeates so many decisions relating to environmental protection. The rationale seems to be based on the notion that a nonpersistent pesticide does its job and then immediately, in a puff, dematerializes into nothingness.

On the contrary, all nonpersistent pesticides merely degrade to other chemicals! The only difference is that most of these new chemicals do not have the same pesticidal action as their parent chemicals. These new chemicals may not kill pests, but what is their toxicity to other organisms? What is their fate in the environment? Do they persist? Do they accumulate?

There are a great deal of data to indicate that some degradation products of nonpersistent pesticides have at least as much potential for nontarget damage as DDT. The identities of many of these degradation products are known because one of the requirements for registration of pesticides for commercial use is study of their environmental fate. However, there is absolutely no program for environmental monitoring of persistent products of nonpersistent pesticides. There is no demand from the groups who lobbied so hard to ban persistent pesticides to investigate the potential environmental damage from nonpersistent pesticides. Why? This is a philosophic question worthy of pursuit for anyone truly concerned about protection of the environment.

The need for increased numbers of applications of nonpersistent pesticides could result in an increased environmental burden of degradation products. By forcing a ban on persistent pesticides, environmentalists may very well have created a much larger environmental problem than the problem they perceived as requiring the ban. Time may tell, if someone asks the right questions.

Time has already told us that the switch from persistent to nonpersistent pesticides has greatly increased the number of acute poisonings among farm workers. Cases of acute illnesses from chlorinated hydrocarbon insecticides were virtually nonexistent prior to their ban. The worst problems were cases of skin irritation. When DDT was banned, the use of organophosphate insecticides increased greatly. This increase was accompanied by a large increase in worker poisonings, some so severe as to be lethal. The efforts to protect wildlife had the ultimate effect of producing acute health problems among workers in the agricultural industry. Despite elaborate programs of worker protection—medical surveillance, protective clothing and cleanup, automatic measuring and mixing devices to avoid human contact, restrictions on reentry into treated fields, and so on—poisonings of farm workers by nonpersistent pesticides still occur.

Man-Made Chemicals Are Very Complex

The third attribute of man-made chemicals that presumably makes them undesirable is their complexity. Many synthetic organic chemicals do have very complex structures. The majority of synthetic chemicals are petrochemicals, which simply means that they are derived from petroleum. Petroleum is an organic substance; thus, petrochemicals are organic chemicals. Organic molecules, both natural and man-made, may be very large and complex or small and relatively simple. Organic compounds are those having the element carbon in their structures. The combination of carbon atoms with atoms of other elements, primarily hydrogen and oxygen, gives rise to an extremely large group of compounds containing many subgroups with widely varying properties and uses. The orientation of the component atoms to each other is an important factor in determining the properties of the individual carbon compounds. All organic compounds, whether natural or synthetic, tend to be much more complex than inorganic compounds because of the nature of the carbon bond.

Some of the most complex chemicals that exist are those produced by living organisms, such as enzymes, hormones, and the DNA molecules that carry genetic information. Some of these natural compounds have been synthesized in whole or in part in the laboratory, but most of them still defy man's skill at chemical synthesis. In fact, many natural organic compounds are so complicated that even the details of their structures still remain hidden. Like nature, man has also synthesized some very complex organic compounds, among which are the polymers, pharmaceuticals, and pesticides mentioned earlier. The complex creations of both man and nature may or may not be toxic. On the other hand, there are many relatively simple inorganic chemicals, such as cyanide and arsenic compounds, all of which may occur naturally or be synthesized in the laboratory, that are much more toxic than complex synthetic compounds such as the drug, aspirin, or the pesticide, malathion. Complexity and toxicity are independent properties of chemicals.

It is essential to an understanding of what makes chemicals toxic to recognize that the degree of toxicity of chemicals does not correlate in any way with whether they are natural or synthetic, biodegradable or nonbiodegradable, simple or complex. Arguments to the contrary, no matter how eloquent the presentation, have no basis in fact and serve only to confound the public.

2

HOW CHEMICALS
CAUSE HARM

Toxicity is just one of the many ways by which chemicals can cause harm. Yet public concern about chemical exposures relates almost solely to the toxic properties of chemicals. The purpose of this chapter is to help broaden that view by describing briefly the other harmful properties of chemicals. A recognition of the fact that chemicals present many different kinds of dangers is essential to protect against human or environmental damage from exposure to chemicals.

HARMFUL PROPERTIES OF CHEMICALS

Explosiveness and Reactivity

Some chemicals are explosive when subjected to physical impact or high temperatures, when they come into contact with air or water, or when they are placed in combination with other chemicals. Explosions, depending on their severity, can cause injury or death as a result of physical or thermal damage to our bodies.

Chemicals that are inherently explosive are not usually found in home settings, but certain chemicals that have a potential for explosion when placed under pressure are found in homes. Some of these chemicals are found in the ubiquitous aerosol canisters that dispense a wide variety of products—foods, hair sprays, pesticides, and so forth. The propellants used in spray cans are gases under ordinary conditions. When placed in pressurized containers they become liquid and occupy a great deal less volume than they do in the gaseous state. When pressure is released by pressing the nozzle, they return to gas form, expand rapidly, and carry the product with them. Under normal conditions of use, aerosol products present little hazard of explosion, but if treated carelessly they can become little bombs or missiles. Aerosol cans should never be subjected to sharp impact, punctured, placed near a high heat source, or left for long periods in strong sunlight. Heat makes gases expand. This greatly increases the pressure inside the container, which can result in an explosion.

Other chemicals that present explosive dangers not generally recognized by the public are found in pressurized gas cylinders. For example, propane cylinders are commonly found in home settings. Some are designed for use with propane torches and others are used with home barbecue grills. Pressurized gas cylinders are also found in hospitals, laboratories, and industrial settings. All pressurized gas cylinders should be handled with extreme care to avoid high temperatures and sharp impact. They should be secured properly during storage and use. They are an especial danger in a fire.

Some chemicals are dangerous because of their chemical reactivity. For example, granular hypochlorite swimming pool chemicals are strong oxidizers. These chemicals can react spontaneously and cause a fire if they contact oils or other combustible materials. In a fire, oxidizing chemicals make all other materials burn more violently. All swimming pool chemicals should be handled and stored with appropriate care.

Examples of chemicals that produce a different type of danger as a result of their reactivity can be found among common household products. Mixing chlorine bleach and household ammonia, a relatively frequent occurrence, can produce very harmful gases know as chloramines. Chloramines have a very low solubility in aqueous solutions; thus, they bubble out of solution rapidly when bleach and ammonia are mixed. Another dangerous combination is chlorine bleach and vinegar. The acid in vinegar causes rapid evolution of chlorine gas. The labels of household products will warn of incompatible combinations if they exist. The label of every home product should be read and understood before use.

Flammability and Combustibility

The distinction between flammable and combustible is based on ease of ignition. Flammables ignite at lower temperatures than combustibles. The Department of Transportation (DOT) uses the distinction for labeling of materials in transport.

Some chemicals are flammable and will burn when they come into contact with a spark or flame at room temperature. Gasoline is an example of a highly flammable liquid. All of the petroleum distillates, such as kerosene, naphtha, and the various hydrocarbon solvents, are either flammable or combustible. They should be handled and stored in a manner that keeps them away from heat and flames.

The chlorofluoro hydrocarbon propellants, used in most aerosol cans until recently, are not flammable, but their replacements may be. Concern about the effects of chlorofluoro hydrocarbons on the ozone layer in the upper atmosphere has led to their replacement by other gases. Some of these, such as propane and butane, are flammable. The caution statement on the product label should tell if the propellant is flammable. If it is, protection should be taken against the flammability hazard as well as the explosion hazard. It is important that no spray stream contacts a lighted cigarette, pilot light, or other flame. Flammable chemicals cause injury or death as a result of tissue destruction from thermal burns.

Radioactivity

In addition to their chemical properties, elements may also be radioactive. Such elements may be naturally occurring or man-made. Because such elements retain their chemical properties they can react to form radioactive chemical compounds that have the same chemical properties as their counterpart, nonradioactive chemical compounds. Small numbers of atoms of practically every chemical element are radioactive. An example is potassium. It is not commonly thought of as having a radioactive form, but about 0.01 percent of all the potassium on earth is radioactive. For all practical purposes, only a relatively small group of chemical elements is classed as radioactive. These have atomic numbers higher than 82 and do not occur in a nonradioactive form. Some commonly mentioned examples of this group are uranium, radium, and radon gas.

Radioactive chemicals cause damage primarily by emission of subatomic particles or rays known as alpha particles, beta particles, and gamma rays. These emissions can alter biochemicals that they strike within cells. The damage done depends on the molecules that are altered. Interactions with DNA molecules can produce mutations (see Chapter 9). Radioactive chemicals act biochemically the same as any other chemical. They may enter the body, where they may be metabolized, excreted, or stored depending on their chemical properties. They are particularly dangerous inside the body, because radiation emitted by these chemicals can directly damage cells and tissue. A good example is radium. Body metabolic processes will store radium in bone tissue. Stored radium continuously bombards adjacent bone tissue. Studies of luminous watch dial painters who through job exposure ingested small amounts of radium show that radiation from the stored radium resulted in leukemia, a form of cancer.

The sources of exposure to radioactive chemicals can be placed in four groups:

1. Naturally occurring radioactive elements, such as uranium, radium, and radon
2. Medical application for diagnosis or treatment, such as radioactive iodine cocktails for study of thyroid function
3. Products of nuclear reactions, such those from nuclear power plants or nuclear explosions
4. Miscellaneous industrial or research uses, such as use of radioactive compounds as biochemical markers in the study of metabolic fate of chemicals

Radioactivity from external sources, such as X-ray machines or other radiation sources, can also be harmful. The important point is that external sources present different problems and risks than the internal sources in the form of radioactive chemicals. Protection against external sources may be accomplished with shielding and safe distance. Protection against internal sources requires protection against the entry into the body of radioactive materials from contaminated air, water, food, and environment. The biochemistry and physics of radioactive materials are subjects that are too complex to be adequately dealt with here. People who want more information can obtain reference materials from a local library.

There has been a great deal of publicity in recent years about the presence of radon in homes and other buildings. Radon is a radioactive gas that is given off by soil, rocks, and building materials made from them, such as concrete and stone. The source of radon is radioactive decay of uranium, which is distributed throughout the earth's crust. The amount of radon emitted from the earth varies with kind of rock formation present and with geographical location. Granites and shales contain more uranium than other kinds of rocks and, thus, emit more radon. The radon accumulates in buildings because structures restrict ventilation. Radon does not accumulate and present a hazard in outdoor air.

The known adverse effect from exposure to radon and the radioactive decay products (RDPs) formed from it is lung cancer. People who want more information about detecting and controlling their radon exposures in homes or workplaces should contact their regional office of the Environmental Protection Agency (EPA) for pertinent booklets.

Corrosiveness

Some chemicals are corrosive and do damage by destroying tissues that they contact. They can destroy skin, but are especially destructive to eyes, mucous membranes of the mouth and throat, and linings of the lungs, esophagus, and stomach. Examples of common corrosives are sodium hydroxide (caustic soda, lye), potassium hydroxide (caustic potash), hydrochloric acid (muriatic acid), and sulfuric acid (oil of vitriol). Corrosive chemicals, like flammable chemicals, cause injury or death as a result of tissue damage. The difference between the two is that corrosives cause chemical burns, whereas flammable chemicals cause thermal burns.

Irritation

Some chemicals are irritants. They do not destroy tissues as do the corrosives, but they produce varying degrees and combinations of redness, swelling, blistering, burning, or itching sensation. Dilute solutions of corrosives, many solvents and polishes, liquids with a low or high pH (acidity or alkalinity), turpentine, pine oil, and spices such as nutmeg, cinnamon, pepper, mustard, and clove are examples of irritants. As a general rule, skin contact with irritant chemicals does not cause death or permanent injury as a result of irritant properties; however, their effects can be very discomforting, both physically and cosmetically. On the other hand, inhalation of irritant gases, such as nitrogen oxides, or irritant fumes, such as cadmium oxide, can cause pulmonary edema which in turn can be fatal.

Sensitization and Photosensitization

Some chemicals can harm us by causing a sensitization reaction. Sensitization is an allergic response. The subject of allergy, which is a subdiscipline of the science of immunology, is much too complex a topic to be dealt with adequately in this chapter. However, because allergy is one of the more common mechanisms by which chemicals cause harm, this chapter must include a brief, if oversimplified, description of sensitization.

Chemicals that cause sensitization are called allergens (or antigens). A single exposure or, in some cases, several repeated exposures to an allergen by inhalation, skin contact, or ingestion may cause the body of the person exposed to manufacture antibodies that will react with the allergen. Once antibodies are formed, the person is sensitized. After a person is sensitized, any future exposure to the allergen, even in amounts very much smaller than the original sensitizing dose or doses, results in an allergic reaction. Allergies may manifest themselves by such symptoms as dermatitis, hives, red or puffy eyes, sneezing, runny nose, headache, and asthma, singly or in combination.

As indicated, sensitization is a response by the immune system. The complexity of immune system reactions is demonstrated by the fact that another response, immunization, involves a sequence of events similar to that of the sensitization response. However, unlike sensitization, which causes illness, immunization protects against illness. Immunization is the process whereby protection against harmful microorganisms, such as smallpox, measles, influenza, or rabies, is obtained. In immunization, harmful organisms (antigens) that have been rendered incapable of causing symptoms of disease but not incapable of being recognized by the body's immune system are injected into the body. The body in turn makes antibodies against the antigen. Once antibodies are formed, the person is immunized. Any future exposure to the harmful organisms results in a reaction between the organisms and the antibodies. This reaction kills or inactivates the organisms and disease is prevented. Immunization may be considered an appropriate response of the immune system and sensitization an inappropriate response. A more complete explanation of the immune system may be found in *In Self-Defense* by Steven B. Mizel and Peter Jaret (see the Suggested Reading section).

It is probable that any chemical, natural or synthetic, is capable of causing an allergic reaction in some individual somewhere in the world, but there are some chemicals that cause sensitization in a significant number of the people with whom they come in contact. Examples of such substances are pollens of all varieties, poison ivy, poison oak, orris root, epoxy resin components, and formaldehyde. Orris root was used many years ago as a base for face powder until its allergenic properties were recognized. Formaldehyde has long been recognized as a sensitizer in occupational settings, but it was not known that it was a problem for the general public until its identification as a component of indoor air pollution (see Chapter 13). People who are sensitive to formaldehyde should know that permanent press clothing may contain trace amounts of formaldehyde that remain as a residue from the treatment process. A few washings should remove this residue.

For most people sensitization is an annoyance and a discomfort, but for some people it is very debilitating and may even result in radical changes in work, life-style, or place of residence in order to avoid trace exposures to the offending allergens. Fortunately, deaths from an exaggerated allergenic response (anaphylactic shock) are rare.

Sensitization must be distinguished from irritation, which it can mimic, particularly when the skin is involved. Irritation and sensitization can both manifest themselves as a dermatitis. Irritants can also produce the same eye symptoms as allergens if rubbed in the eye or chest symptoms if the irritant is inhaled. Irritation is a purely local or topical phenomenon, whereas sensitization is a systemic condition. Only a physician can determine if symptoms are allergic in nature.

Photosensitization is a similar phenomenon, except that light is required to trigger the adverse reaction. Photosensitization may occur as a result of oral, dermal, or inhalation exposure. The photosensitization reaction has several manifestations. There may be hivelike swellings, acnelike eruptions, severe sunburn, or a combination of the three in areas of the skin exposed to light. With repeated episodes of photosensitization, the affected skin may develop a permanent darkening and be more subject to skin cancer. Examples of chemicals that can cause photosensitization are coal tar compounds, such as creosote and dyes derived from them; some forage plants, such as St. Johnswort and buckwheat; and a number of drugs, such as phenothiazine, aureomycin, and sulfonamides.

Toxicity

Finally, many chemicals can cause harm by virtue of their toxicity. Toxicology is the science that investigates the adverse systemic effects of chemicals. The mechanisms by which a chemical exerts a toxic action are many and varied. Some chemicals are themselves toxic. Others must be converted metabolically to other forms before they become toxic. Some chemicals may damage any cells or tissues with which they come in contact. Others damage only one specific kind of cell or tissue. Some chemicals act directly on cells or tissues. Others act indirectly in some manner, such as by interfering with some biochemical reaction, altering some physiological mechanism, or destroying an essential nutrient, which in turn is the damaging event. Regardless of the mechanism, the principles that govern the harmful property of chemicals known as toxicity apply equally to all chemicals, both natural and synthetic.

The toxicity of a chemical refers to its ability to damage an organ system, such as the liver or kidneys, or to disrupt a biochemical process, such as the blood-forming mechanism, or to disturb an enzyme system at some site in the body removed from the site of contact. This is in contrast with corrosiveness, which does damage at the site of contact. The systemic damage that chemicals do is not capricious or random. A chemical does not affect one set of functions in one person and a different set in another. If it did, its effects would be unpredictable, and there could be no such thing as a science of toxicology. A chemical can have an effect on several different functions within an individual, and individuals can vary among themselves with regard to the sensitivity of their different functions. Thus, for example, it may appear that a chemical affects the kidneys in one person and the liver in another, but clinical examination will reveal the liver and kidney involvement in both.

Every chemical has some set of exposure conditions in which it is toxic and, conversely, every chemical has some set of exposure conditions in which it is not toxic. Hopefully, the chapters that follow will make this very difficult concept comprehensible.

Multiple Harmful Properties

Some chemicals may possess only one of the above harmful properties, whereas others can produce damage by several means. For example, hydrochloric acid and sodium hydroxide are corrosive in concentrated form and irritants in dilute solution. Neither is classed as toxic, that is, they do not cause damage at a site removed from the site of contact, but both can cause death by destroying tissues they touch. In such cases, death is the result of the body's inability to survive the harm caused by tissue destruction. In contrast, hydrofluoric acid, a relative of hydrochloric acid, is not only very corrosive but also very toxic.

Gasoline, while extremely flammable, has a relatively low toxicity. It presents a unique danger when ingested if some of the liquid is aspirated. Gasoline and all other petroleum distillates, when taken into the lungs in liquid form, will produce a chemical pneumonitis. The fatality rate from petroleum distillate pneumonitis is quite high. For this reason, household products that contain 10 percent or more of petroleum distillates must carry a warning not to induce vomiting if ingested. The act of vomiting greatly increases the chances that some of the material will be aspirated. Petroleum distillate pneumonia is seen most frequently in children who drink furniture polish. However, adults also can become very seriously ill or die as a result of accidentally aspirating gasoline, such as can occur while siphoning it from an automobile gas tank.

The only other chemicals that are required by law to carry a "Do not induce vomiting" warning on the label are the corrosives. With corrosives, the danger is not chemical pneumonitis, but rather the chance that the act of vomiting will subject a corroded esophagus to sufficient stress to cause esophageal rupture.

DEFINITION OF POISON

A chemical that causes illness or death is often referred to as a poison. This concept is erroneous and has resulted in a great deal of confusion in the public mind about the nature of the toxic action of chemicals. Poisons are chemicals that produce illness or death when taken in very small quantities. Legally, a poison is defined as a chemical that has an LD_{50} of 50 milligrams (mg), or less, of chemical per kilogram (kg) of body weight. An LD_{50} is the quantity of a chemical administered in one dose that is lethal for 50 percent of the test animals within a 14-day period. LD means lethal dose and the subscript 50 refers to the percentage of the animals for which the dose was lethal. Chapter 7 describes the LD_{50} more fully.

Fifty mg/kg is equal to approximately three-fourths of a teaspoon for an average adult and about one-eighth of a teaspoon for an average 2-year-old child. There are very few chemicals that are lethal in such small quantities. Thus, there are not many chemicals that can be classed as poisons, yet there are many, many chemicals that are capable of causing illness or death. Even among the dreaded pesticides, the majority do not fall within the category of poison. Therefore, to consider that only poisons are harmful or that harmful chemicals are, of necessity, poisons is a misleading and dangerous oversimplification.

LD_{50}'s are almost always related to the toxicity of chemicals; however, chemicals that are corrosive can also kill, especially when they are ingested. Thus, a corrosive chemical, like a toxic one, will be classed as a poison if it is lethal in doses of 50 mg/kg or less. A good example of chemicals that are labeled as poisons because of their corrosiveness are the well-known drain-opener products that are found under almost every kitchen sink. One might consider it splitting hairs to distinguish between corrosiveness and toxicity as a cause of death. Although the distinction has little significance in human terms, it is one that must be made in a proper study of the harmful effects of chemicals.

DEFINITION OF HAZARD

Another distinction that should be made is the difference between toxicity and hazard. The latter has come into common use as a synonym for the former. Actually hazard is a much more complex concept than toxicity because it includes conditions of use. The hazard presented by a chemical has two components: (1) the inherent ability of a chemical to do harm by virtue of its explosiveness, flammability, corrosiveness, toxicity, and so forth; and (2) the ease with which contact can be established between the chemical and the object of concern. These two components together describe the chance or probability that a chemical will do harm. For example, an extremely toxic chemical, such as strychnine, when sealed in an unopenable vial, can be handled freely by people with no chance that a poisoning will occur. Its toxicity has not changed, but it presents no hazard because no contact can be established between the chemical and people. Conversely, a chemical that is not highly toxic can be very hazardous when used in a manner that makes it readily available for accidental ingestion.

For example, boric acid is not very toxic acutely but is very hazardous when used as a component in boric acid roach tablets. Boric acid is a very effective roach killer. When applied in powder form in spaces behind cabinets and under drawers where it is inaccessible, it presents no hazard at all, but it can be very hazardous when combined with sugar and formed into tablets that are scattered around baseboards. A young child crawling around the kitchen floor can find and eat these tablets without being observed. Several hours later, when symptoms appear, the cause will not be known and the urgency of getting medical attention will not be recognized. The fatality rate for accidental boric acid intoxication in children is about 50 percent.

3

TOXICOLOGY—A
BRIEF HISTORY

Toxicology is the study of the adverse systemic effects of chemicals. All substances that caused illness or death were originally referred to as poisons. Today, the more general term *toxicant* is used, with *poison* being reserved for the special class of toxicants that require only very tiny amounts to cause death. A toxicant is now defined as a chemical that does systemic damage, but the word came originally from the Greek words *toxon* and *toxikos*. These words referred to bows and arrows used for hunting game. Early cultures found that their bows and arrows were more effective if the arrows were dipped in toxic juices obtained from plants. Arrows coated with toxic juices would kill or immobilize the victim. If an arrow did not kill the animal or bird (or enemy), it could escape capture. The possibility that traces of arrow toxins might be present in the flesh of meat apparently did not concern primitive hunters. Meat obtained in such a manner today would probably not be accepted by the public, even if it did meet current regulatory requirements.

EMPIRICAL TOXICOLOGY

Empirical toxicology, as distinguished from the science of toxicology, predates recorded history. Prehistoric man knew which poisonous plants and animals to avoid from seeing the sad experiences of his fellow beings. These experiences also told him which plant juices to use as toxins for his arrows. The fact that certain substances could cause acute illness or death was known to even the most primitive of human populations because it was so obvious—the cause–effect relationship was so direct.

Before the beginnings of recorded history a large number plant and animal toxins were recognized. The early Greek physicians catalogued many toxins—animal, plant, and mineral. As civilization progressed, so did the art of poisoning. Empirical toxicology became applied toxicology. Notable historic examples of the application of toxicology are the execution of Socrates by means of a hemlock brew, the suicide of Cleopatra by means of a bite of an asp, and the many political assassinations of medieval times by means of a variety of plant and mineral toxicants.

Empirical toxicology is concerned almost exclusively with the acute toxicity, the immediate toxicity, of chemicals. The fact that substances could cause chronic intoxication—illness or death from long-term, low-level exposure to chemicals—was not recognized until relatively recently in the history of man. The first hints that chronic exposure to chemicals could cause illness came from occupational exposures. Mercury and lead were among the first chemicals to be suspect.

The poorer health of people who worked at certain trades, particularly those involving manual labor, such as mining, metallurgy, or the making of pottery, was noted by early Greek and Roman physicians. Hippocrates described severe colic in men who extracted metals, which he attributed to lead poisoning. Pliny wrote of mercury poisoning among slaves who worked in the quicksilver mines of Almaden, Spain. But in those days, manual laborers and slaves were considered to be inferior beings who lived unhealthy life-styles; therefore, their poor health was not considered remarkable. They suffered a high background incidence of disease, physical infirmity, and deformity caused by accidents, abuse, and the stresses of poverty. The diseases caused by the chemicals to which they were exposed blended into the background incidence and were hidden. It was not for another 1,500 to 2,000 years that the connection between disease and chronic exposure to chemicals would be given serious consideration.

PARACELSUS AND RAMAZZINI

In 1567 the first monograph on occupational diseases of miners and smelters was published, 26 years after the death of its author, the Swiss physician Paracelsus. In his monograph, Paracelsus distinguished between acute and chronic toxic effects of metals, and described in detail the symptoms of chronic mercurialism.

Paracelsus was a man far ahead of his time, a bridge between alchemy and science. He was an iconoclast with a contempt for the medical doctrines and methods of the day. Thus, he earned the disdain of the medical establishment, which led to numerous moves of his medical practice. However, he was an itinerant physician probably as much by choice as by necessity. Though disliked by his peers, Paracelsus was extremely popular with his students and patients, among whom were counted members of many of the ruling families of medieval Europe.

Paracelsus lectured and wrote not in Latin, which was the custom of the time, but in his native German. He preferred the company of laborers, tradespeople, gypsies, and others unacceptable to genteel folk. He died at the age of 48 as a result of wounds suffered in a tavern brawl in Salzburg. In his short span of years he set the stage for a revolution in medical practice by teaching his student physicians to use chemical medications rather than the more popular magic potions.

Paracelsus set forth one of the basic tenets of modern toxicology when he wrote: "What is it that is not poison? All things are poison and nothing is without poison. It is the dose only that makes a thing not a poison." Testimony to this truth is found in Paracelsus' own writings. He not only was the first to publish a description of the symptoms of chronic mercury poisoning but was also the first to design a rational chemotherapy using mercury for the treatment of syphilis. Paracelsus' treatment was used until the discovery of the arsenic compound arsphenamine (Salvarsan) by Paul Ehrlich, a German bacteriologist, more than 350 years later.

Since the awareness that chemicals could be chronically toxic was born in the study of the diseases of occupations, no discussion of the origins of that awareness would be complete without mention of Bernadino Ramazzini, who is considered to be the father of occupational medicine.

Ramazzini was born in Italy in 1633 and lived to the age of 81, active in his profession until the end. Ramazzini's specialty was epidemiology, the study of the incidence, prevalence, and movement of diseases in a population—diseases that attack many people in a region at the same time. He was also a very socially oriented physician who had noted the wretched conditions of workers in the trades. He felt that medicine should strive to improve the quality of life of the common people.

Ramazzini was once told by a sewer worker that a man who had never done such work could not possibly understand what it was like. Ramazzini took this admonition to heart. In all of his studies of the occupations he followed his subjects into the mines, factories, and cesspools to see and experience the conditions under which they labored. He learned that there is no substitute for firsthand knowledge and that occupational exposures could be involved in the causation of disease. Ramazzini is remembered today by the medical profession for his wise counsel that, in addition to the usual questions, doctors should inquire into the occupations of their patients.

PHARMACOLOGY—TOXICOLOGY

Pharmacology (from the Greek, *pharmakon,* a drug) is one of the oldest of the biological sciences. It is defined as the study of the action of drugs, their nature, preparation, administration, and effects. Substitution of the word *chemicals* for *drugs* in the definition would give a more appropriate description of the early science. The whole universe of known chemicals came under the scrutiny of early pharmacists in their search for substances that had healing effects. All substances were considered to be potential candidates for medicinal use. Thus, the pharmacology literature is replete with information on beneficial and adverse effects of a tremendous number of naturally occurring chemicals, both organic and inorganic, that are not classed as drugs in modern usage of the term.

The development of synthetic organic chemistry freed pharmacologists from some of their dependence on nature's bounty and enabled them to tailor-make drugs to fill specific therapeutic needs. Modern pharmacology, which developed along with modern medical science during the nineteenth and early twentieth centuries, has added many synthetic chemicals to its list of drugs and deleted most of the old-fashioned remedies from its inventory of medicinal preparations.

The science of toxicology, as contrasted with empirical toxicology, is a young science compared to many other biological sciences. It was born of pharmacology and, until relatively recent years, was considered a subdivision within the science of pharmacology. Pharmacology, of necessity, embraced toxicology because it is neither possible nor practical to study only therapeutic effects to the exclusion of toxic effects. In fact, the relationship between toxic effect and therapeutic effect forms the basis for an extremely important medical concept—the therapeutic index. The therapeutic index of a drug is the number obtained by dividing the dose that is toxic by the dose that gives the desired curative effect. The larger the therapeutic index (the greater the difference between the dose that harms and the dose that helps), the safer the drug.

Early interest in the toxic effects of chemicals was directed toward symptoms of acute poisoning, methods of treatment of poisoning victims, and later to the legal aspects of criminal cases. The early Egyptian and Greek physicians recorded the effects of many poisonous plants and substances derived from them. Application of this knowledge became a way of life among the ruling Italian families during the fifteenth century. During the Renaissance, the act of poisoning was developed into a fine art. It was practiced on relatives, friends, and political rivals. *Borgia,* the name of the notorious family that helped perfect the art, has become synonymous with *poisoner.*

Impetus for the study of toxicology, as a separate science from pharmacology, came primarily from occupational medicine. The first systematic classification of all of the chemical and biological information available at the time was published in the early nineteenth century by M. J. B. Orfila, a Spanish physician who taught at the University of Paris. History credits

Orfila with being the first to consider toxicology as a discipline separate from pharmacology.

The rapid growth of the synthetic organic chemical industry during the past several decades brought with it a greatly heightened awareness and concern about the toxic action of chemicals. The science of toxicology is now fully recognized as a discipline separate from pharmacology.

REGULATION OF TOXIC CHEMICALS

The regulation of toxic chemicals in the United States predates by many decades current demands for control of synthetic chemicals that enter the environment. In the late nineteenth and early twentieth centuries, publicity about gross contamination and adulteration of foods that resulted from industry malpractices created a public demand for reform of the food industry. In addition, the public became concerned about chemicals that were added, either deliberately or inadvertently, to canned and packaged foods.

During the same period, Harvey W. Wiley, chief of the Department of Agriculture's Bureau of Chemistry, was a vocal advocate of wholesome, unadulterated food. During the last quarter of the nineteenth century, Dr. Wiley and his staff studied the composition of foods and their adulterants. He was quoted as saying in 1902, "There has been too much argument about the effects of chemical preservatives on health. I propose to find out by scientific experimentation what is the truth about a question of such vital concern to consumers of the nation. Some day we will have a law" (Linton, F. B., Federal food and drug leaders, *Food Drug Cosmetic Law Quarterly* 4:451–470, 1949). Dr. Wiley's prophecy came to pass when, after more than 20 years of consideration of similar measures by Congress, the Pure Food and Drug Act of 1907 was enacted. Administration of the Act was placed in the Bureau of Chemistry, and Dr. Wiley was appointed the first Food and Drug Commissioner. His task was not easy. The Food and Drug Commissioner had authority to investigate, but little power to enforce. Dr. Wiley and his assistants, known as the poison squad, made many political and industry enemies. However, it was too late to still public interest and awareness of the problem of contaminated and adulterated foods and drugs.

In 1910, the Federal Insecticide Act was passed. It was the government's first attempt to control the sale and use of insecticides. The legislation did not stimulate much enforcement activity because there were so few insecticides available for use by agriculture. One of the most commonly used insecticides was the very toxic lead arsenate. Cases of accidental poisoning and acute illnesses among applicators from lead arsenate, combined with concerns about chronic health effects of lead arsenate residues, kept interest in toxic chemical regulation alive, if relatively inactive, in the minds of legislators and regulators.

Two important events took place in 1927. First, increasing public demands for pure foods and drugs resulted in the creation of the Food and Drug Administration (FDA) to administer the Pure Food and Drug Act. All responsibility for the Act was transferred from USDA to FDA. For the first time since 1907, an organization existed for the sole and specific purpose of enforcing pure food and drug laws.

The second important regulatory event of 1927 was passage of the Federal Caustic Poison Act. The many tragic deaths and disfiguring, disabling injuries among children who swallowed lye (sodium hydroxide) provided the stimulus for passage of this Act. Soap making was a common household chore for women of the time, particularly in rural communities. Lye, a necessary ingredient to make soap, was commonly found in cabinets accessible to small children. The Act, which was primarily a labeling law, was an attempt to protect children from corrosive materials by requiring warning labels on such products. The labels informed adults of the dangers of ingesting these materials. Theoretically, the adults, in turn, would store the labeled products out of the reach of children.

Over the next years, few changes were made in the food, drug, and insecticide laws. A major regulatory action usually occurs only after a disaster or public demand requires it. Such was the case with the enactment of the Food, Drug, and, Cosmetics Act (FDCA) of 1938. Congress had been at work for years on measures to strengthen the 1907 Act. The elixir of sulfanilamide tragedy of 1937 (see Chapter 7) provided the extra bit of incentive required for passage of a stronger and more protective law than the 1907 Act.

Despite many decades of public concern about the safety and purity of foods and drugs, the modern era of toxic chemical regulation did not begin until after World War II. Legislation regulating toxic chemicals has for the most part followed public concerns. As mentioned above, laws affecting foods, food additives, and cosmetics were passed in the first part of the twentieth century. After World War II, concurrent with the rapid development of the synthetic pesticides, laws were passed to control both their use and their residue levels in food. The public, legislators, and regulators recognized that advances in pesticide technology, with the tremendous increase in numbers of pesticides available and their volume of use, required increased public and consumer protection. The Federal Insecticide, Fungicide, and Rodenticide Act (FIFRA), enforced by USDA, was passed in 1947, and the Miller Amendment to the FDCA, enforced by FDA, was passed in 1954. In 1958, the much-publicized Delaney Clause, the amendment that prohibits the use of any food additive that is found to induce cancer when ingested by man or animal, was added to FDCA. The provisions of FIFRA and FDCA supplemented each other. They provided uniformity in requirements for toxicity testing, tolerance-setting procedures, and so on for the chemicals under their respective purviews.

During the 1950s and 1960s there was a steady increase in legislation regulating a wide variety of chemicals that enter homes, workplaces, and the general environment. During this period, public interest was expanded to include air and water pollution. A series of laws were passed to control automobile exhaust emissions and industrial discharges to both air and water. At about the same time, the need for environmentally sound methods for disposing of household, commercial, and industrial refuse became increasingly important. Problems associated with dumps that included environmental damage, air pollution, ground and surface water pollution, and public nuisance have resulted in a series of laws to recycle, treat, store, and dispose of both chemical and household waste.

Concern for the health and safety of children also held the attention of the public. In 1960, the much more broad Hazardous Substances Labeling Act (HSLA) superseded the Caustic Poison Act of 1927. HSLA, like the Caustic Poison Act, was a child-protection measure. It applied to all products sold for home use, or products that could conceivably be brought into homes because of small container size that are not covered by other laws, such as foods, drugs, pesticides, and cosmetics. HSLA, like the Caustic Poison Act, was only a labeling law. It defined many more categories of hazards associated with household products and specified labeling for each. The Act was based on the assumption that parents will read labels and take appropriate steps to protect their children. HSLA was strengthened in 1970 by the Poison Prevention Act. This Act required that child-proof containers be used for products considered to be too hazardous for labeling alone to be effective in protecting children.

The EPA came into being in December 1970. Rachel Carson's book *Silent Spring* (Boston: Houghton Mifflin), published in 1962, stimulated public awareness of environmental chemicals, particularly pesticides. During the years that followed, the public became increasingly fearful that pesticides and other chemicals were harming them, their loved ones, and the environment. The decision to bring regulation of the many kinds of environmental chemicals together in one agency, stimulated by public concerns about toxic chemicals, resulted in the creation of the EPA. Essentially all control over pesticide use was taken from USDA and FDA and placed in EPA. In addition, EPA was given jurisdiction over a wide variety of other chemicals that had a potential for environmental pollution, for the purpose of protecting wildlife and the environment.

In the 1960s and 1970s, interest also began to focus on chemicals used in industry and the impact of these chemical uses on workers and on the neighborhoods surrounding individual plants. Expanding knowledge and awareness of chemical hazards provided a stimulus to industry for self-regulation. As a result, this period saw increased development of guidelines for procedures and practices to protect workers in chemical and related industries.

The first legislative action in response to the interest in worker health was the Occupational Safety and Health Act of 1970. Responsibility for its enforcement was placed in a new agency, the Occupational Safety and Health Administration (OSHA), located in the Department of Labor (DOL). The Act is a worker protection law designed to prevent traumatic injuries as well as occupational diseases. It addresses the whole issue of job-induced injuries, including health hazards and their control. Its passage finally gave official recognition to the long-known fact that the people at greatest risk from exposure to toxic chemicals are the people who work with them.

One of the most important new ideas to come out of this law was the Hazard Communication Standard promulgated by OSHA. The Hazard Communication Standard, also called the worker right-to-know law, requires manufacturers and importers of chemicals to determine the hazards of each product they sell. They are also required to transmit the hazard information and associated protective measures to their employees and customers through labels and material safety data sheets (MSDS's). Employers, in turn, are required to make MSDS's available at the job site and to inform workers about the nature of the hazards involved and how to protect themselves. Workers have the right to see and study these data sheets.

The right of people to know about the chemicals in and around their own communities was brought into focus in December 1984 by the chemical plant disaster in Bhopal, India. Operating problems at this chemical plant resulted in the release of thousands of pounds of methyl isocyanate, a toxic and very corrosive gas, without warning into the nearby city of Bhopal. Approximately 2,000 people were killed and 30,000 were injured. After studying this accident and other plant disasters, the U.S. Congress passed the Emergency Planning and Community Right-to-Know Act of 1986. Among other important provisions, this law requires plant owners to notify specified government agencies of chemical inventories, and chemical releases to air, water, and waste disposal facilities. It also requires plant owners to provide a chemical inventory list and copies of MSDS's to local fire departments. Under the law, all of these data are available to the public.

The two decades since the creation of EPA and OSHA have seen numerous amendments to and refinements of the many laws regulating toxic chemicals. Some of the laws regulating exposure to chemicals recommend or require that standards be set for such exposures. As a result, there are numerous sets of standards for permissible acute and chronic exposure to chemicals. Some are promulgated by public agencies and carry the full force of law. Others are merely recommendations or guidelines proposed by public or private organizations. Standards are named by the agency or act that establishes them. For example, standards for food additives and pesticide residues in foods are called tolerances. Standards for chemicals in potable water are called drinking water standards. Standards for chemicals in ambient air are called national ambient air quality standards. Standards for chemicals in the air in occupational settings are called permissible exposure limits.

The public should be aware that the existence of a standard does not necessarily mean that the chemical is present in the permitted quantity. For that matter, it may not even be present in any quantity. The need for this caveat became apparent many years ago when DDT was making daily headlines. It was generally known that a tolerance of 7 ppm DDT (parts of DDT per million parts of food) was permitted in certain specific foods for which a tolerance had been requested. Logically, the public assumed that all foods, not just those for which a tolerance had been granted, contained 7 ppm DDT. In actual fact, monitoring by federal and state agencies demonstrated that DDT could be detected only in a fraction of the permitted foods, and almost invariably in concentrations well below 7 ppm.

A major concern of many people is pesticide residues that are present in foods. The FDA conducts routine monitoring of pesticide and other chemical contaminants in more than 100 different food items, representing 11 or more different food groups, collected from retail markets throughout the United States. Adult diets have been monitored since 1960 and infant and toddler diets have been monitored since 1974. The results of these studies, called "Total Diet Studies" or "Market Basket Surveys," are published regularly in the *Journal of the Association of Official Agricultural Chemists.*

Several private agencies also monitor pesticide residues in foods. A study of residues in California produce conducted by the Natural Resources Defense Council (NRDC) in 1984 showed trace quantities of one or several different pesticides in 44 percent of samples tested. Almost all of the pesticide residues found were between 10 and 30 percent of the tolerances set by the federal government. These results are not significantly different from those reported by FDA in their market basket surveys.

Although monitoring programs indicate that pesticide residues in fruits and vegetables grown in the United States are well within the tolerances set by EPA, there is considerable public concern that the monitoring programs themselves are inadequate. There is even more concern that imported produce is not subjected to the same scrutiny as domestic produce. Public confidence is further eroded when pesticides are misused and result in excessive residues in some food product. Fortunately, although well publicized, such episodes are not common.

The public's concerns about pesticide residues in foods have resulted in the creation of a new and unofficial regulatory mechanism. A number of produce markets and supermarket chains have hired private analytical laboratories to test their produce. Such private testing programs permit markets to assure the public that there are no (or no significant) quantities of pesticides present on their fruits and vegetables. Consumers may consider the comfort provided by such an effort is worth the cost. However, its benefit to public health is considered by regulators to be of little or no significance because, as mentioned above, routine monitoring by state and federal agencies shows no or very low levels of pesticide residues in domestic produce.

The public is generally unaware of how much time, effort, and money are expended in developing and monitoring standards designed to protect its health. Instead, the average person seems to feel that no one cares, and is usually quite surprised when informed of the standards that do exist. There are some who will deny that anyone does care, or who will contend that efforts to protect the public health are grossly inadequate. Such perceptions are subjective and can be argued as passionately and sincerely as their counterpositions. Actually, the question of degree of involvement by government in protecting public health is one that society must answer. How much is it willing to risk, and how much is it willing to pay? Regardless of whose name is on the bill, it is always the consumer who pays.

The history of regulation of harmful chemicals in the United States over the past 100 years has been the response of one government to the problems that arose out of the growing use and importance of chemicals. Early on, the concern was for chemicals and impurities in food and drugs. As uses grew and more chemicals were developed, laws were passed to control pesticide use and pesticide residues. With continued growth, the need was to deal with the more complex problems of environmental pollution, waste disposal, occupational exposures, neighborhood risks, and the right to know. One of the most recent problems relating to toxic materials is their presence in waste disposal sites and their migration into groundwater. The Superfund Amendments and Reauthorization Act (SARA) was passed in 1986 to hasten the cleanup of hazardous waste sites.

History has also shown that laws have changed and evolved with time to meet changing needs, changing perceptions, and changing costs. The laws have also been changed by the great and rapid improvements in the sciences of toxicology and analytical chemistry. This process of change will no doubt continue for as long as required by the needs of society.

A list of many categories of substances regulated by various federal agencies, although by no means complete, is given in Appendix D. In some instances, regulation involves standard setting and enforcement; in others it specifies manufacturing, processing, testing, or handling procedures, labeling, reporting of certain kinds of information, or record keeping. Appendix D will provide key words that the reader can use to obtain further information about any product from a public library, college or university library, or from the agency responsible for regulation of the product.

4

FACTORS THAT INFLUENCE TOXICITY: HOW MUCH— HOW OFTEN

All effects of chemicals—beneficial, indifferent, or toxic—are dependent on a number of factors. The most important factor is known as the dose–time relationship: how much chemical is involved (dose) and how often during a specific period of time the exposure occurs (time). The dose–time relationship gives rise to two different types of toxicity that must be distinguished from one another: acute toxicity and chronic toxicity. The acute toxicity of a chemical refers to its ability to do systemic damage as a result of a one-time exposure to relatively large amounts of the chemical. Acute toxicity is the concern, for example, when children are exposed to some household product left within their reach, or when some substance is accidentally spilled during transportation and passersby or neighborhood residents are exposed. The exposure is sudden and often becomes an emergency situation.

Chronic toxicity refers to the ability of a chemical to do systemic damage as a result of many repeated exposures, during a prolonged period of time, to relatively low levels of the chemical. Chronic toxicity is the concern in the evaluation of the health impact of food additives, pesticide residues, or the effects of exposure to chemicals encountered by working people during the normal course of their employment. If chronic exposure to a chemical is of sufficient magnitude to produce adverse effects, such effects are usually not detected until the exposure has continued for some period of time.

ACUTE VERSUS CHRONIC TOXICITY

Why must acute and chronic toxicities be distinguished from each other? Because the symptoms produced by these two extremes of exposure usually bear no relationship to each other. Chronic toxic effects cannot be predicted from a knowledge of the effects produced by acute exposures; the two extremes of exposure usually involve different organ systems or different biochemical mechanisms. The corollary that acute effects cannot be predicted from a knowledge of chronic effects would also hold true. However, such a need never arises because knowledge of acute symptomatology of a chemical always proceeds and surpasses that for chronic poisoning (intoxication). Acute effects of chemicals are much more readily apparent and much more easily studied than chronic effects.

To illustrate the lack of relationship between acute and chronic effects, the symptoms of acute intoxication by sublethal quantities of chlorinated solvents, such as chloroform or carbon tetrachloride, are primarily those of the central nervous system—that is, excitability, dizziness, and narcosis. Chronic symptoms are primarily those of liver damage. Symptoms of acute arsenic intoxication refer mainly to the gastrointestinal tract, with vomiting and profuse and painful diarrhea. Chronic intoxication produces skin changes and damage to the liver, peripheral nerves, and the blood-forming mechanism. Acute symptoms of lead intoxication are mainly gastrointestinal. Chronic symptoms are those that result from damage to the blood-forming mechanism, nervous system, and muscular system.

Obviously, between the two extremes of acute toxicity and chronic toxicity there are an infinite number of combinations of quantity (how much) and frequency (how often) of exposure. Frequent exposure to relatively large amounts of a chemical can produce features of both acute and chronic symptomatologies. Adverse effects from these latter kinds of exposure are referred to as the subacute toxicity of a chemical.

Not only do the symptomatologies of acute and chronic intoxication by a given chemical bear little relationship to each other but neither do their relative potencies. A chemical that is highly toxic acutely is not necessarily highly toxic chronically and, conversely, a chemical that is of a low order of toxicity acutely is not necessarily low in toxicity chronically.

Before proceeding further, LD_{50}, a term first mentioned in Chapter 2 and commonly used to describe acute toxicity, should be explained further. LD means lethal dose, and the subscript 50 means that the dose was acutely lethal for 50 percent of the animals to whom the chemical was administered under controlled laboratory conditions. A subscript of 0 would mean that the dose was lethal for none of the animals and a subscript of 100 would mean that the dose was lethal for 100 percent of the animals. The units of the LD_{50} are mg/kg, which means milligrams of chemical per kilogram of body weight of animal. The LD_{50}'s of chemicals with low to moderate toxicity are usually given in grams per kilogram (g/kg) rather than mg/kg. The smaller the LD_{50}, that is, the fewer the milligrams of chemical per kilogram of body weight required to kill the animals, the greater the acute toxicity.

Conversely, the larger the LD_{50}, the lower the acute toxicity. LD_{50} and acute toxicity are inversely related. A more complete discussion of the LD_{50} concept will be presented in Chapter 7.

There are some chemicals that are very highly toxic acutely, but chronically in very small amounts they are not toxic and may even be essential. Vitamin D is an example of such a chemical. Vitamin D, in pure form, is highly toxic acutely, with an oral LD_{50} of about 10 mg/kg, or 400,000 International Units per kilogram (IU/kg). The organophosphate pesticide, parathion, also has an oral LD_{50} of about 10 mg/kg. If vitamin D were not exempted from the Hazardous Substances Labeling Acts (both federal and California) by virtue of its being a food (when present in milk or other food) or a drug (when sold as a vitamin), in pure form it would be required to carry a poison label (LD_{50} of 50 mg/kg or less). Yet, despite its very high acute toxicity, each one of us requires an average of 10 μg (400 IU) of vitamin D every day for good health. Vitamin D deficiency results in the disease known as rickets. Severe deficiency can cause death. Vitamin D can be chronically toxic when taken in daily doses several times greater than 400 IU. Daily doses of more than 2,000 IU (five 400-IU capsules per day) should be taken only under medical supervision.

People who take vitamin D supplements need not be concerned about the very high acute toxicity of the vitamin D they purchase in capsule form without a prescription. It is so tremendously diluted that each capsule contains only a recommended daily dose. For example, an acutely lethal dose of 400-IU vitamin D capsules for a young child would exceed 10,000 capsules (400,000 IU/kg body weight ÷ 400 IU/capsule × 10 kg body weight = 10,000 capsules).

Sodium fluoride is another example of a chemical that is highly toxic acutely, but essential in trace amounts. It has an oral LD_{50} of about 35 mg/kg. Chronically, in very small amounts of 1 or 2 mg daily, it is essential for good dental health. In quantities of 3 or 4 mg per day or greater, sodium fluoride can cause mottling of tooth enamel in some young people whose permanent teeth are in the formative stages. Larger daily quantities can produce chronic fluorosis, a condition characterized by increased bone density and spurring.

People who are opposed to fluoridation of domestic water supplies take issue with the claim that the practice is safe and essential to protect the dental health of the public. The fact is that numerous and extensive epidemiologic studies of people who have lived for a lifetime in areas that have water supplies with a naturally high fluoride content show no effects attributable to fluoride, other than mottled teeth and fewer cavities. A slight increase in bone density was found in people with the highest fluoride intake, a finding not unexpected in light of the known interference by fluoride in the metabolism of calcium, an important element in bone composition.

However, further study indicated that this increased density was of no medical significance. In fact, a current treatment for the severe osteoporosis associated with menopause that is meeting with some success is oral administration of fluoride salts in quantities that approximate those ingested by people with the highest naturally occurring concentrations of fluoride in water. Natural fluoride waters contain up to 8 milligrams per liter (mg/l), which would give a daily dose of 8 to 16 mg fluoride per day.

Sodium chloride, common table salt, is another chemical that is acutely toxic, but daily, in very small amounts, it is essential for life. Salt has an oral LD_{50} of about 3 g/kg. If salt were not excluded from the Hazardous Substances Labeling Act because it is a food, it would be required to be labeled with a caution that it might be harmful if swallowed (LD_{50} from 50 mg/kg up to 5 g/kg). There have been deaths among children who have been given a box of salt to play with, or who have gotten into the saltcellar and ingested a lethal quantity of salt. A lethal dose of table salt for a 1-year-old child would be about 2 tablespoons. Chronically, table salt is toxic to people who have heart or kidney disease. In addition, excessive use of salt has become recognized in recent years as a causative or contributing factor in some cases of high blood pressure. Yet small amounts of salt daily are essential for life.

It has long been considered that the critical part of the salt molecule is the sodium atom, which is provided for adequately in the normal diet; however, recent studies indicate that the salt molecule itself (sodium chloride) might be the culprit in some cases of high blood pressure. It has been estimated that, under ordinary environmental conditions, the minimum requirement for adults is about 200 mg of sodium per day. People who work or live in very hot environments and experience excessive sweating may require larger amounts of salt to make up for the salt lost in sweat. By careful selection of low-sodium foods and by eliminating the use of salt in cooking and at the table, the intake of sodium can probably be reduced to between 1,000 and 2,000 mg per day, an amount well above the basic requirement. The average American diet is well laced with sodium, to the extent of 8,000 to 10,000 mg daily. A person on a low-sodium diet should recognize that many dietary components other than salt furnish sodium; monosodium glutamate, sodium citrate, and sodium bicarbonate are just a few examples.

In contrast to chemicals that are acutely toxic and chronically nontoxic, there are some that are just the reverse—acutely nontoxic and chronically toxic. Metallic mercury is one such chemical. A one-time ingestion of large amounts of metallic mercury will not cause illness or death. Thus, the frantic mother whose child chews on the thermometer and swallows the mercury contents need have no fear: The mercury will be eliminated in the feces. It will cause no harm because the amount of mercury absorbed from the intestinal tract is very small. But if a child swallowed the contents of a thermometer every day over a long period of time, the small amount of mercury absorbed each day could give rise to chronic mercury intoxication. Metallic mercury must not be confused with mercury salts. The latter are very toxic both acutely and chronically.

The pesticide cryolite (aluminum sodium fluoride) is another chemical that does not cause acute illness or death. The largest quantity of cryolite that can be ingested at one time will not produce illness. The cryolite passes through the intestinal tract and is eliminated without adverse effect. But if animals are fed cryolite every day in their feed, they soon become ill and die. Cryolite is a very insoluble compound; the small amount of chemical that is absorbed from a one-time exposure is not sufficient to cause illness, but absorption of the same small amount every day, day after day, can cause chronic illness and death. As a general rule, chemicals that are insoluble or only slightly soluble tend to be nontoxic or of low toxicity acutely.

A chemical that is considered completely nontoxic, acutely and chronically, is water—the fluid of life. But there are a few rare cases reported in the medical literature of both acute and chronic intoxications, some even fatal, from excessive water intake. Quantities considered excessive would be measured in gallons per day. Death from drinking excessive amounts of water occurs as a result of literally drowning the cells and tissues of the body.

Most chemicals have some degree of both acute toxicity and chronic toxicity, but there is no way that one can estimate how toxic a chemical will be chronically solely from data on the degree of acute toxicity. Despite the general lack of correlation in severity between acute and chronic toxicities of chemicals, the effects of both acute toxicity and chronic toxicity are dose-related, that is, the greater the dose, the greater the effect.

SIGNIFICANCE OF DIVIDED DOSES

The tremendous importance of the dose–time relationship in determining whether or not a chemical will be toxic is well illustrated by the fact that every one of us ingests many lethal doses of many chemicals, both natural and synthetic, during the course of a lifetime. A shocking thought! But consider, there is a lethal dose of caffeine in approximately 100 cups of strong coffee. There is a lethal dose of solanine in from 100 to 400 pounds of potatoes. There is a lethal dose of oxalic acid in 10 to 20 pounds of spinach or rhubarb. There is a lethal dose of ethanol in a fifth of scotch, bourbon, gin, vodka, or other hard liquor. A listing of foods that contain potentially toxic chemicals would fill many pages. If all or even most of these foods were eliminated as food sources, people would suffer or die from malnutrition.

How can we ingest so many lethal doses of so many chemicals and yet survive? We survive because we do not take in 100 cups of coffee all at one time, or 100 pounds of potatoes, or 10 pounds of spinach, or a fifth of liquor. We take our poisons in divided doses—not all at one sitting. Our bodies can handle small amounts of foreign chemicals, both natural and synthetic. We metabolize them or excrete them unchanged without their doing any damage. In fact, there are data in the toxicology literature that indicate that our bodies are not just indifferent to trace quantities of foreign chemicals, both natural and synthetic, but that such exposures may actually be beneficial. As a general rule, with the exception of toxicologists who study the chronic toxicity of chemicals in mammalian systems, scientists and health officials are unaware of these data due to their lack of familiarity with the toxicologic literature.

The concept that exposure to trace quantities of foreign chemicals may actually produce beneficial effects is unacceptable to some people. They reject evidence supporting the concept by labeling it the result of artifacts in experimental data. But rejection cannot change the fact that the phenomenon exists, and its frequency of occurrence suggests that it is not due to artifacts. The concept of *sufficient challenge,* the name given to the phenomenon by Dr. H. F. Smyth, Jr., many years ago, will be explored more fully in Chapter 8.

All living organisms, since the beginning of time, have had to deal with exposure to numerous noxious substances. No animal on earth could survive a day, much less live to reproduce future generations, if it were not capable of handling small amounts of a wide variety of foreign chemicals. It is only when we overwhelm the natural defense mechanisms of our bodies, by taking in too much at one time, or too much too often, that we get into trouble.

5

FACTORS THAT INFLUENCE TOXICITY: ROUTE OF EXPOSURE

The degree of toxicity of a chemical is dependent not only on the dose-time relationship, as discussed in Chapter 4, but also on its route of exposure. The route of exposure is the pathway by which a chemical enters the body. There are three principal routes of exposure: (1) penetration through the skin, (2) absorption through the lungs, and (3) passage across the walls of the gastrointestinal tract. These routes are labeled dermal, inhalation, and oral, respectively. Thus, by combining the dose-time and route factors, six kinds of toxicity can be identified for every chemical: acute dermal, acute inhalation, acute oral, chronic dermal, chronic inhalation, and chronic oral toxicities.

Chemicals can enter our bodies by other routes, but they are of little practical significance for the average person. A chemical may be injected into a vein (intravenously), into a muscle (intramuscularly), into the skin (intradermally), under the skin (subcutaneously), or into the peritoneal cavity (intraperitoneally). All of these routes are commonly used to study the physiology, pharmacology, and toxicology of chemicals in animal species, but human exposure by these routes is encountered only in medical practice, or in cases of self-inflicted substance abuse.

PRINCIPAL ROUTES OF EXPOSURE

Dermal

Probably the most common way of contacting chemicals is by the dermal route. Fortunately, intact skin is an effective barrier against many chemicals. If a chemical cannot penetrate the skin, it cannot exert a toxic effect by the dermal route. If a chemical can penetrate the skin, its dermal toxicity depends on the degree of absorption that takes place. The greater the absorption, the greater the potential for a chemical to exert a toxic effect.

As a general rule, the majority of inorganic chemicals are not absorbed through intact skin. Organic chemicals may or may not be absorbed, depending on a number of conditions. Usually, an organic chemical in dry powder form is absorbed to a lesser degree than the same chemical in an aqueous solution, suspension, or paste. An oily solution or paste permits greater absorption than an aqueous vehicle. Certain solvents, such as dimethyl sulfoxide (commonly known as DMSO), greatly enhance the dermal absorption of a wide variety of compounds. Chemicals are absorbed much more readily through damaged or abraded skin than through intact skin. Once a chemical penetrates the skin, it enters the bloodstream and is carried to all parts of the body.

Inhalation

Inhalation is a second common route of exposure to chemicals. Unfortunately, unlike the skin, the surface of the lungs is a poor barrier against the entry of chemicals into the body. In addition, we have a great deal more lung surface than skin surface. It has been estimated that the average adult has about 20 ft^2 of skin and about 750 ft^2 of lung surface. Because of the extremely important job that the lungs have to do, namely transfer oxygen from air to blood and carbon dioxide from blood to air, that 750-ft^2 area of lung surface is a very delicate thin membrane, in large part only one cell thick, that separates the air in the lungs from the blood in the tissues of the lungs. This delicate thin membrane allows ready passage to the bloodstream not only of oxygen but also of many other chemicals that may be present as contaminants in inhaled air. This direct access explains why people smoke marijuana rather than eat it. It gives them a greater and more rapid high. It also serves as a good example of the dependence of effect on route of exposure.

In addition to systemic damage, chemicals that pass through the lung surface may also injure its delicate, vulnerable membrane and interfere with its vital function. Chemicals such as asbestos and materials that contain crystalline silica, such as quartz dust, cause disease by damaging lung surfaces. These diseases are known as asbestosis and silicosis. Asbestos also can cause cancer in the lung and in other sites. There are a number of other materials that damage lung surfaces, such as cotton dust and coal dust. These diseases are all grouped together under the heading of pneumoconioses.

If a chemical cannot become airborne, it cannot enter the lungs and, thus, cannot be toxic by the inhalation route. Chemicals can become airborne in two ways, either as little tiny particles composed of many molecules or atoms (dust, mists, or fumes) or as individual molecules or atoms (gases or vapors). Solids that have a low vapor pressure do not become airborne to any great extent as individual molecules, but they can be ground into very fine particles and become dispersed into the air as dusts.

Dust particles become respirable only when they are below a certain very small size. The largest of the respirable particles deposit on the surfaces of the nasopharynx or throat and, thus, do not enter the lungs. Smaller particles are breathed into the lungs and impinge on the lung surfaces. As the particles become even smaller, a certain percentage of them remains airborne even in the alveolar spaces. Particles that remain airborne are breathed in and out with the respiratory movements. Some of these airborne particles do, by chance, hit the bronchial or alveolar walls and remain in the lungs for a period of time. Vapors and gases, which are present in air as individual molecules or atoms, are also breathed in and out with the respiratory movements. The number that impinges on the walls of the respiratory tract and the lung surfaces is dependent on their concentration in air.

Inhaled particles that do not dissolve in the fluids coating the lung surfaces may lodge in the lungs for a long period of time, perhaps even permanently, or they may be swept back up the lung passages by cilial action and eliminated from the body by coughing. The latter is the more common occurrence. Cilial action is reduced in smokers who inhale, which may account in part for smoker's cough. Excessive coughing may be an attempt by the body to compensate for the less effective action of the cilia. If we did not have efficient lung clearance mechanisms, those of us who live in dusty environments would soon have our lungs filled solid, a circumstance obviously incompatible with life. Chemicals that are absorbed through the surfaces of the lungs enter the bloodstream and are distributed to other parts of the body by the general circulation.

Oral

The third way that chemicals enter our bodies is by ingestion. The oral route is the principal pathway for entry of substances that are present in foods. Chemicals that are ingested enter the body by absorption from the gastrointestinal tract. If they are not absorbed, they cannot cause systemic damage. Absorption of chemicals can occur anywhere along the digestive tract, from the mouth to the rectum, but the major site for absorption is the small intestine. Nitroglycerine, for example, can be absorbed through the mucous membranes of the mouth; hence its medicinal administration by placement under the tongue to relieve the pains of angina pectoris. Some chemicals, such as ethyl alcohol, are absorbed from the stomach as well as the small intestines. That is why the effects of alcoholic beverages are felt so rapidly and why food in the stomach can help delay those effects.

Absorption from the stomach occurs to a much greater extent in infants than in adults. In addition, infants up to the age of about 9 months have gastric juices that are alkaline in pH rather than acidic, as they are in adults. This physiologic difference is considered to be the reason why nitrates, which are present in some well waters, are so much more toxic to infants than adults. Alkaline gastric juice enhances the activity of microorganisms that reduce nitrates to their very much more toxic nitrite form.

Some chemicals are absorbed through the walls of the rectum; thus, certain drugs can be administered in the form of rectal suppositories. This is particularly advantageous when the oral route is not practical or possible. A number of chemicals can be absorbed from the large intestine, although the major function of this segment of the gastrointestinal tract is absorption of just one chemical—water. The small intestine, located between the stomach and the large intestine, is the major site for the entrance into the body of all of the absorbable substances that we eat, which, of course, are primarily foods. Chemicals absorbed from the small intestine follow one of two paths. As a general rule, water-soluble chemicals go directly from the small intestine to the liver via the hepatic portal vein. Fat-soluble chemicals bypass the liver by going into the lymphatic system, which empties into the bloodstream near the heart.

Combinations

In actual practice, it is difficult to have an exposure to a chemical that is solely by the dermal, inhalation, or oral route. Dermal exposure can also become ingestion exposure when hands are not washed after handling or working with chemicals and before eating or smoking. Inhalation exposure can also become ingestion exposure when some of the chemical deposited on the walls of the nasopharynx is swallowed along with the secretions from that cavity, or when it is coughed up from the lungs and swallowed. Thus, when route of exposure is specified, what really is meant is exposure primarily, rather than solely, by that route.

INFLUENCE OF ROUTE ON TOXICITY

There are a few chemicals that are equally toxic by all three routes of exposure. The organophosphate pesticide parathion is an example. It is highly toxic acutely by skin absorption, inhalation, and ingestion. Parathion, like other organophosphates, exerts its toxic action by inhibiting cholinesterase enzymes, regardless of how it enters the body. Cholinesterase enzymes are biochemicals that our bodies use to deactivate other biochemicals known as choline esters. Acetylcholine is a choline ester that serves as a biochemical mediator of nerve impulse transmission. When cholinesterase is inhibited, acetylcholine is not deactivated and, as a result, there is a continued stimulation of the parasympathetic nervous system. Symptoms of parasympathetic stimulation, such as excessive salivation and pinpoint pupils, then appear. Death can ensue as a result of too great a depletion of cholinesterase activity.

Repeated exposures by any route to levels of parathion that do produce acute symptoms may eventually result in changes in phosphate resorption by the kidneys or in electroencephalographic changes. There have been no reports of obvious clinical effects resulting from chronic exposure to parathion at concentrations that produce no change in normal cholinesterase values. On the other hand, studies with other organophosphate compounds have shown behavioral and neurological changes in people chronically exposed to concentrations that do not produce clinical symptoms (Weiss, Bernard, Neurotoxic risks in the workplace, *Applied Occupational and Environmental Hygiene* 5(9):587–594, 1990).

The majority of chemicals are not equally toxic, acutely or chronically, by all three routes. Vitamin D, which is highly toxic acutely by mouth, is essentially nontoxic acutely and chronically by the dermal route. Vitamin D requirements can be met by skin application, but hypervitaminosis D (vitamin D overdose) cannot be produced by this route. Nothing is known about the inhalation toxicity of vitamin D, but since it does not become airborne under ordinary conditions, the inhalation route is of no practical concern.

Metallic mercury is not considered to be acutely toxic by any route, but it is chronically toxic by ingestion. Mercury vapors are very toxic by inhalation. As mentioned in the previous chapter, a child who swallows mercury from a thermometer will not be harmed, but a child who breaks the thermometer and lets the mercury fall into the pile of the bedroom rug, or into a crack in the floor, may be in danger. Metallic mercury is a volatile liquid—it is readily converted from the liquid form to the vapor form. The degree of risk from spilled mercury depends on the concentration of mercury vapor reached in the air, which in turn depends on how much mercury is spilled, the temperature of the room, and the amount of air circulation present.

People at particular risk from mercury vapor intoxication are those who use metallic mercury in their occupations. Mercury vapors are a significant occupational hazard for personnel who work with silver amalgam fillings in the dental profession (Schneider, M., *J. Am. Dental Assoc.* **89**:1092, 1974). Thus, it is absolutely essential to observe good housekeeping procedures when working with metallic mercury in order to avoid chronic exposure to its vapors. Metallic mercury should never be stored in uncovered containers.

If mercury is spilled, it should be cleaned up immediately, no matter how small a quantity is involved. Metallic mercury is a very heavy liquid, almost 14 times heavier than water, and it has a much greater tendency to stick to itself than to anything else, with the exception of other metals such as gold or silver. Thus, when cleaning up spills it is important to either wear gloves or to remove all rings. If you do not, you may find that your gold rings or other jewelry have turned a silvery color where they were touched by the mercury. The mercury has formed an amalgam with the gold and may cause damage to the metal.

When mercury spills, it usually spatters into many small droplets. If the amount of metallic mercury spilled is larger than the quantity that would be in a thermometer, the local health department should be consulted for advice and help in decontamination, particularly if the mercury has gotten into rugs or cracks in the floor. Spilled mercury can present such a serious inhalation hazard that home vacuum cleaners should never be used to collect mercury droplets. Vacuum cleaners, unless specifically designed for hazardous waste removal, increase the air concentration of mercury by causing more rapid and complete vaporization of the droplets.

To clean very small spills in a home situation, a small wooden stick such as a toothpick can be used to gently tease the droplets toward each other so that they coalesce into larger droplets. Then the larger droplets can be rolled into a glass or plastic vial that has a stopper or a cap. This can be a very tedious process, but it is an essential one. Since metallic mercury is not acutely toxic, there is no need to worry about exposure during a cleanup process. The stoppered vial of mercury should be put away in a safe place until the next visit to a dentist. The mouth washbasins in dentists' offices are now equipped with traps that collect gold, silver, and mercury for recycling. A dentist can easily dispose of small quantities of mercury.

Periodically, the fact that silver amalgam fillings contain metallic mercury is rediscovered. The attendant publicity raises concern that people are being poisoned by their dental fillings. Numerous studies have been conducted over the years to evaluate the possibility of mercury toxicity from dental amalgams. Despite anecdotal reports to the contrary, there is no evidence that people with dental amalgam fillings suffer toxic effects. For a period of about a week after a silver amalgam filling is inserted (or removed) urinary excretion of mercury is slightly elevated. However, the effect is transient and well below levels consistent with mercury intoxication. Although dental amalgams are not associated with chronic toxic effects, the possibility that they may cause allergic reactions exists. Fortunately, cases of hypersensitivity to mercury are rare.

There are two basic reasons why toxicity varies with route of exposure.

One relates to the quantity of chemical that gains entry into the body and the other to the pathway that the chemical follows in its course through the body. Assuming the pathway to be of no influence, a chemical will be most toxic by the route that permits it greatest entry. As a general rule, the lungs offer the least resistance to the entry of chemicals. Many chemicals can gain entry through the intestinal tract, although there are some chemicals that are poorly absorbed or not absorbed by this route. The skin provides the best barrier of the three routes. For example, a chemical readily absorbed through the lung surfaces but poorly absorbed through the skin would be more toxic by inhalation than by dermal exposure. Conversely, a chemical that penetrates the skin more readily than the lungs (a rare circumstance— I am not aware of the existence of any airborne chemical that would fit in this category) would be more toxic by the dermal route.

The influence of pathway through the body on the toxicity of chemicals is a very much more complex matter than degree of absorption. It is dependent not only on the sequence in which tissues and organs are reached by the chemical but also on the physiologic and metabolic events that occur along the way. It also depends on where target organs (those damaged by the chemical) fit in the scheme.

Ingested chemicals may be worked on by intestinal microorganisms to yield products that are more toxic, less toxic, or of the same toxicity as the parent compound. These products may or may not be absorbed from the intestinal tract in the same manner and degree as the parent compound. Thus, the oral toxicity of a chemical may differ from its dermal or inhalation toxicity merely by virtue of its passage through the intestinal tract.

The majority of compounds absorbed from the small intestines go first to the liver, via the hepatic portal vein, before entering the general circulation of the body. The liver is the great metabolic factory of the body. It plays a major role in the body's metabolic conversions, not only of biochemicals but also of foreign chemicals. Foreign chemicals may be converted by the liver to compounds of greater toxicity, lesser toxicity, essentially the same toxicity, or they may not be metabolized at all. After residence in the liver, any of the chemical that remains unreacted and its products enter the bloodstream to be circulated to all other parts of the body. Thus, assuming equal absorption by the oral, dermal, and inhalation routes, a chemical converted to a less toxic form by the liver would be less toxic by ingestion than it would by inhalation or skin absorption because it is detoxified by the liver before it goes to other tissues or organs. The converse would be true if the liver converted the chemical to a more toxic form.

Some chemicals that are absorbed into the body from the small intestines bypass the liver by going into the lymphatic system rather than into the hepatic portal vein. The lymphatic system carries them back toward the heart where they enter the bloodstream and then are carried to all other parts of the body. Chemicals that follow this liver bypass are primarily fat-soluble compounds, such as fatty acids, fat-soluble vitamins, and some of the large-molecule synthetic organic compounds. These chemicals are not acted upon by the liver before being distributed to other organs. Thus, their toxicity is not immediately affected by passage through the liver.

Chemicals absorbed through the skin or lungs are sent directly to all other organs of the body before going to the liver, at least during their first excursion around the circuit. There may be some metabolic conversion during this passage but, if it occurs, it is usually to a much lesser degree than the conversions that occur in the liver. The molecules of a compound that are not excreted by the kidneys, skin, or lungs soon after absorption will eventually find their way to the liver. Once they reach the liver, they are treated in the same manner as if they had gone to the liver directly.

All chemicals that enter the body are transported in the bloodstream. The network of blood vessels that winds through all tissues and organs is the body's delivery system, and the blood is the transport medium. Its major function is to carry nutrients to every cell and carry away waste products. All foreign chemicals that enter the body are also carried around in the bloodstream until they are disposed of by excretion, metabolism, or storage.

ROUTES OF ELIMINATION (EXCRETION)

All foreign chemicals that enter the body eventually exit from the body, either in the same form as they entered or after being metabolized to other compounds. The three routes of entry considered in this chapter are also routes of exit; however, the kidneys and lungs are the major organs for excretion of chemicals from the bloodstream. The kidneys might be considered the sewage treatment plants of the body. They scavenge the blood and filter out the major portion of dissolved solids. However, they are more discriminating than sewage treatment plants in that they then selectively return essential (and some not so essential) substances to the blood. Metabolic waste products, excess biochemicals, and the majority of water-soluble foreign compounds are eliminated from the blood in urine produced by the kidneys.

The gas carbon dioxide and other metabolic products that are easily converted to gas or vapor form are excreted through the lungs. Many gases, such as anesthetics, that are absorbed into the body from the lungs are also excreted in large part, or solely, by the lungs. Small organic molecules that enter the body by other routes may also be excreted through the lungs. A well known example of the latter is ethyl alcohol. Shortly after imbibing an alcoholic beverage, small quantities of alcohol begin appearing in the breath. This is the basis for the much contested breath test for drunk driving.

There are other minor routes for excretion of chemicals. One is the skin. Small quantities of water or oil-soluble compounds leave the body in sweat or oil gland secretions, respectively. Another is the bile duct. The bile, produced by the liver, serves as a vehicle for excretion of some fat-soluble chemicals. Bile empties into the small intestine via the bile duct, from whence the compounds excreted in the bile may be absorbed back into the system or eliminated in the feces. Reabsorption of foreign compounds after biliary excretion greatly complicates studies of storage and excretion of fat-soluble chemicals.

6

OTHER FACTORS THAT INFLUENCE TOXICITY

The two previous chapters have shown that both dose–time relationship and route of exposure exert a profound influence on the acute and chronic toxicities of chemicals. In addition, there are a number of other factors that modify toxicity. These include species, age, sex, nutrition, state of health, individual sensitivity, the presence of other chemicals, the phenomenon known as adaptation, and possibly light. With the exception of species, the degree of influence that these factors possess is not readily apparent or well investigated. However, there are sufficient data from controlled animal experiments or from human experience to demonstrate that they each are capable of exerting some degree of influence on the toxicity of at least some chemicals.

SPECIES

The fact that species differ in their responses to the toxic properties of chemicals is of great practical significance to toxicologists. The science of toxicology depends heavily on data obtained from animal experimentation for its judgments about the toxicity of chemicals for humans. Species differences must always be carefully evaluated when using data obtained from animal experiments to estimate potential human toxicity.

There is a great deal of information in the scientific literature concerning differences among species in their sensitivity to chemicals. For example, methanol, also known as wood alcohol, is very toxic acutely and chronically, by ingestion and inhalation, for humans and other primates. It is much less toxic for all other species, and no other nonprimate species suffers the ocular damage and blindness that is produced in humans by methanol intoxication. Another example is the industrial chemical tri-*ortho*-cresyl phosphate, or TOCP. Acute or chronic exposure, by all routes, to TOCP demyelinates nerve fibers in humans and chickens, but not in dogs or rats. Myelin is a biochemical that serves as a protective coating for certain kinds of nerve fibers. Demyelinization is the destruction of this protective sheath. Demyelinization can result in a polyneuritis, progressing to paralysis, which may or may not be reversible, depending on the degree and duration of intoxication.

Another chemical that also shows marked species difference is nitrobenzene, which converts hemoglobin to methemoglobin (an oxidized form of hemoglobin that is incapable of serving the oxygen transport function of hemoglobin). Nitrobenzene and related chemicals are more toxic acutely and chronically by all routes to humans, cats, and dogs than they are to monkeys, rats, and rabbits. The latter do not respond to nitrobenzene exposure with any significant degree of methemoglobin formation.

The list of chemicals that have different toxicities for different species is extremely long and could be the subject of many volumes. The reasons for such variations are often elusive. When a mechanism is revealed, it is most often found to be due to the fact that species handle the compound in a slightly different manner: They absorb, metabolize, or excrete it to a greater or lesser extent, or at a faster or slower rate. Differences among mammalian species in metabolism of foreign chemicals are usually quantitative rather than qualitative. They are usually differences in degree rather than differences in kind. Animal species possess essentially the same metabolic pathways for handling most chemicals. The end product of metabolism depends on which of the pathways is used.

Quantitative differences occur when different species metabolize a chemical utilizing the individual pathways to different degrees. Qualitative differences occur when entirely different pathways are used for metabolizing the same chemical. Mammals are very similar in the metabolic pathways they possess within the cells of their bodies. However, the degree to which they use one biochemical pathway rather than another for the metabolism of a given chemical can vary widely.

Occasionally a difference is due to some physiologic peculiarity. For example, rats are unable to vomit. Thus, when a rat ingests a toxicant, it is unable to expel the material from its stomach. The inability to vomit prevents the rat from eliminating the toxicant before it does damage. Dogs, on the other hand, can voluntarily eject the contents of their stomachs. Most dog owners are quite familiar with the heaving motions that a dog utilizes to induce vomiting when it has ingested some offending substance. The inability to vomit, peculiar to rodent species, accounts for the apparently greater acute oral toxicity of some compounds for the rat as contrasted with the dog and other nonrodent species. Such chemicals are ideally suited for use as rodenticides.

Variations in toxicity of chemicals with species are of great practical importance because almost all of the knowledge of adverse effects of chemicals is obtained from toxicologic testing procedures in laboratory animals. These procedures are conducted almost entirely for the purpose of evaluating the toxicity of chemicals for humans. Thus, laboratory animals are considered to be the animal models or, more properly, surrogates for humans.

Where does the human fit in the scheme of relative toxicity? He does not rank consistently among animal species with regard to sensitivity to chemicals; some chemicals are more toxic for humans than for other animals and some chemicals are less toxic for humans. In fact, there is no mammalian species that will always place in the same rank on listings of relative sensitivity to a series of individual chemicals.

Proximity in the phylogenetic scheme does not assure similarity of response. One would expect that another primate, such as the monkey, would be the most appropriate animal model for the human. This is true for some chemicals, but not for all, as demonstrated by the above references to methanol and nitrobenzene. The monkey responds as the human does to methanol intoxication, but with methemoglobin-formers such as nitrobenzene, monkeys and humans react very differently. Thus, in the case of nitrobenzene, the dog or cat is a more appropriate animal model for the human than the monkey.

There has been a great deal of discussion during the past several decades concerning the extent to which data obtained from animal experimentation can be extrapolated to humans. The view that data from animal experimentation cannot be translated to humans under any circumstances has long had some proponents, particularly among people with an antichemical bias. Such a view demonstrates a basic lack of understanding of the sciences of comparative physiology, pharmacology, and biochemistry and the principles, practices, and procedures of toxicology. If there were absolutely no relationship between humans and other mammals in their responses to chemicals, we would have no methodology for evaluating adverse effects of chemicals or, for that matter, beneficial effects of drugs, nutrients, and so forth, for the human species. The consequences of such a situation for human health and well-being would be incomprehensibly tragic. The billions of dollars spent yearly by government and industry in programs for conducting and evaluating animal toxicity tests would be a useless and unjustified waste.

Fortunately, such is not the case. There are many common threads woven through the fabric of bioevolution. Humans are not unique in their anatomy, physiology, or biochemistry. The similarities among mammals are far more numerous than are the differences. At the molecular level, humans even show a kinship with single-celled organisms in cellular anatomy and biochemistry. For example, one of the final pathways for converting sugars, fats, and some amino acids to their end products of energy, carbon dioxide, and water is the same for almost all living organisms whether they are plants, microorganisms, or animals. This pathway, known as the Krebs cycle or the tricarboxylic acid (TCA) cycle, was first studied in yeasts—the same kinds of organisms that are used to raise our bread and brew our beer.

The proposition that data obtained from animal experimentation can be applied directly and quantitatively to humans is so obviously flawed that it has had no proponents until relatively recently. There is sufficient species variation in the toxicity of chemicals to make a blind transfer of data from animals to humans very dangerous. Many of the recent converts to the direct-transfer thesis are the very same people mentioned above, who have classically maintained that data obtained from animal experimentation could not be used under any circumstances for translation to humans. They adopted the latter position in order to reject any data that indicated there were no adverse toxic effects from chronic exposure to trace quantities of synthetic environmental chemicals. Now, in situations where the effect is cancer and where the data from animal experiments are positive, they maintain that it is appropriate to translate data directly from animals to humans.

The first, and to this date only, legal blessing for the position that data from animals are directly applicable to humans can be found in the much-debated Delaney Clause of the 1958 Food Additives Amendments Act. This clause requires that chemicals used as food additives be considered as human carcinogens if they produce cancer in any animal species, at any level of exposure. It must be stressed here that the Delaney Clause applies only to food additives. During the past 25 years, it has never been extended to any of the many other chemicals in our environment primarily because of objections from the scientific community. With few exceptions, toxicologists reject the concept of the Delaney Clause because it excludes the exercise of scientific judgment in the evaluation of toxicity data.

The opposing views (1) that toxicity data from animals can be transferred directly to humans and (2) that they cannot are both overly simplistic. The extrapolation of animal data to humans requires sound toxicologic judgment.

AGE

There is very little information available from human experience concerning the impact of age on the toxicity of chemicals in humans. It is known that age exerts an influence on the acute oral toxicity of some chemicals in controlled studies in laboratory animals. Newborn or infant animals may be more sensitive than adults to the adverse effects of some chemicals, and less sensitive than adults to other chemicals. For example, DDT is not acutely toxic to newborn rats. It becomes progressively more toxic as the animals mature, until it finally reaches an LD_{50} of 200 to 300 mg/kg in adult rats. The opposite is true with the organophosphate pesticide parathion. Despite its very high acute oral toxicity to adult rats, it is even more toxic to newborn animals. Data from accidental poisonings with parathion indicate that the same is true for the human species. The quantities of parathion that have caused illness or death among children are considerably less than predicted from calculations based on quantities that have caused the same effects in adults. Boric acid is another chemical that seems to be much more acutely toxic orally to human infants and toddlers than to adults.

Differences between young and adult animals in their responses to certain chemicals are considered to be due in part to differences in the activity of the enzyme systems that metabolize foreign chemicals. These systems, known as the liver microsomal enzyme systems, are underdeveloped in immature animals. Thus, a chemical converted to a less toxic metabolite by liver microsomal enzymes would theoretically be less toxic to adults than to infants. The fully developed liver microsomal enzyme systems of the adult would metabolize the toxic chemical more quickly and effectively than the immature infant systems would. Conversely, a chemical converted to a more toxic form by the liver microsomal enzymes would be more toxic to adults than to infants.

Despite the almost complete lack of scientific data on the influence of age on toxicity in humans, claims are now being made that children are more affected by exposures to chemicals than adults. The most recent argument against the use of pesticides in agricultural production, or at least for stricter government control of such use, is that pesticide residues present a particular carcinogenic risk to children. The argument that pesticides are much more damaging to children than to adults has tremendous emotional impact and, superficially, seems very logical. It is offered as a scientific fact rather than merely a theory, which is what it actually is. The rationale for the theory has three major premises:

1. The relative intake of pesticides is greater in children than adults.
2. Growing children, with their more rapidly dividing cells, provide more sites than adults do for attack by carcinogens because dividing cells are more vulnerable to DNA damage than quiescent cells.
3. Children are more sensitive than adults to the toxic effects of chemicals.

An examination of each premise is important to an evaluation of the validity of the theory. First, infants and young children do consume considerably more food per unit body weight than adults. During the early years, the need for energy and nutrients from food for body growth and development is greater than at any other period of life. As the child develops, physical activity increases greatly and adds to the child's energy demands. Thus, if a child consumes relatively more of a food than an adult, and that food contains a pesticide residue, the relative pesticide intake is greater in the child. However, the critical point is not that children ingest relatively greater quantities of pesticides than adults, if they indeed do, but how their exposures relate to levels considered safe, such as Acceptable Daily Intakes (ADIs) set by the World Health Organization (EPA is now using the term RfD or RFD, meaning Reference Dose, to express the same concept as ADI). Data from total diet studies conducted by FDA (see Chapter 3) show that the diets of infants and toddlers contain quantities of pesticides only about one hundredth of their respective ADIs. ADIs, in turn, are set at one hundredth or less of levels considered safe.

The second premise is based on the fact that dividing cells are more vulnerable to DNA damage than cells that are in a resting state. This fact is fundamental to the success of chemotherapy. Tumors grow rapidly because their cells divide often. Normal cells divide much less often than tumor cells. Drugs that are used to treat cancer probably destroy dividing cells by causing mutations in their DNA molecules. At any given time tumors have many more dividing cells than normal tissues, which makes tumors more sensitive to the drugs than normal tissues. By analogy, children, with their more rapidly dividing cells, are more vulnerable to carcinogenic chemicals. During periods of growth, cells divide more often to make more of themselves. In this manner, cell divisions increase the volume of tissues and size of organs.

If rapid growth does, in fact, increase the vulnerability of an organism to carcinogens, pesticides would be low on a list of relative risk. The majority of pesticides have not been shown to be carcinogenic. Among those that have caused cancers in animal studies, the majority do not cause cancer unless they are converted in the body to another chemical that is a carcinogen (see Chapter 10). Many pesticides are metabolized as foreign chemicals by the liver microsomal enzymes, mentioned above. Since immature enzyme systems do not metabolize foreign chemicals efficiently, and hence cannot convert foreign chemicals to a carcinogenic form as readily, children may be more protected than adults from the carcinogenic properties of pesticides. Probably the greatest carcinogenic risk for growing organisms is exposure to ionizing radiation, which can contact DNA molecules directly. For the majority of humans such radiation exposure is from natural sources.

The third premise, that children are more sensitive to toxic effects of chemicals, depends on how the word *sensitive* is defined. If it is used to mean that children are harmed by smaller doses than adults, then children are more sensitive. As explained in Chapter 7, the acute toxicity of chemicals is expressed as milligrams or grams of chemical per unit of body weight. Since the body weight of a child is so much less than that of an adult, the dose of any chemical that would be harmful to a child is proportionately less than the dose that would harm an adult.

However, the word *sensitive* is more often used to mean that chemicals are more harmful to children independent of body weight differences. This is an intuitive concept not supported by scientific evidence. As discussed above, animal studies show that some chemicals are relatively more toxic to the young than to adults and other chemicals are relatively less toxic. There is no evidence that humans are different from other animal species in this regard. Thus, the common assumption that infants are always more sensitive than adults to the toxic effects of chemicals is not scientifically valid. However, since so little is known about the influence of age on toxicity of chemicals in humans, it is a warranted assumption for purposes of regulating chemical exposures.

SEX

The obvious physical and physiologic differences between the sexes relate to their roles in the reproductive process. The fact that exposure, especially occupational exposure, to certain foreign chemicals could have a profound impact on this process has only become generally recognized in recent years. The effectiveness of chemicals as birth control substances has been the subject of research for many decades. It is only in recent years that research efforts have been directed toward revealing unwanted adverse effects on the reproductive process. The subject of reproductive toxicity is discussed in Chapter 11.

Excluding the effects of chemicals on the reproductive process, it is known that sex, per se, does influence toxicity of chemicals in animals. Essentially nothing is known about the differences between men and women in their reactions to toxicants. In laboratory animals, some chemicals display marked sex differences in toxicity, acutely, chronically, or both. For example, male rats are about 10 times more sensitive than female rats to liver damage from chronic oral exposure to the pesticide DDT. Some organophosphate pesticides are more toxic acutely for female rats and mice than for males, whereas the reverse is true for other organophosphate pesticides.

Anatomic and physiologic differences between males and females are dictated by the sex hormones; thus, it is assumed that sex differences in toxicity are also due to hormonal influences. Indeed, there is much indirect evidence in animals to support this thesis. Sex differences in toxicity of chemicals are usually abolished by castration or by hormone administration. In addition, chemicals that do show a sex difference in adult animals often show no such difference in immature animals.

NUTRITION

Diet plays an important role in toxicity of chemicals for laboratory animals. It is assumed that it also modifies the toxicity of chemicals for humans, despite the fact that there is a relative paucity of data on the subject.

As a general rule, diets adequate in proteins and vitamins protect against the toxic effects of chemicals. The simplicity of this rule belies the great complexity of nutrition–toxicity interactions. This complexity is further compounded by data showing that laboratory animals fed diets nutritionally adequate but restricted in quantity, without the addition of any added foreign chemical, develop significantly fewer tumors than animals fed all that they want to eat of exactly the same diet. The subject of nutrition is beyond the scope of this book, but anyone interested in individual responses to nutrients should read the works of Roger J. Williams and Walter A. Heiby (see the Suggested Reading section).

STATE OF HEALTH

A person's individual response to toxicants is influenced by his physical and his emotional health. For example, certain physical conditions, such as liver disease or lung disease, enhance the toxic effects of chemicals that cause liver or lung damage, respectively. Medical experience has shown that table salt and possibly other sodium-containing salts are chronically more toxic to people with heart or kidney disease than they are to people with normally functioning hearts and kidneys. There are very few controlled animal experiments reported in the scientific literature that relate physical health to toxicity of chemicals. However, scientists who conduct animal toxicity studies have long recognized that laboratory animals must be in good health in order to be valid experimental tools. Sick or maltreated animals do not give reliable results.

The impact of emotional health on toxicity of chemicals is an even more difficult subject to study than the influence of physical health. There are convincing data in the medical and dental literature to indicate that various emotional stresses adversely affect physical health. Thus, there is an intuitive sense that they also must exert some influence on toxicity, even if only indirectly. Many articles on the influence of stress on such medical conditions as cancer and allergies have appeared in the popular press in recent years.

BIOCHEMICAL INDIVIDUALITY

The reactions of individuals vary with all of the preceding factors but, in addition, there is a great deal of empirical evidence for the fact that a person's biochemical makeup can also modify the toxicity of chemicals. This factor is referred to as individual susceptibility or biochemical individuality. The most obvious expression of differences among individuals in their reactions to chemicals is seen in their acute responses. There is no such thing as one dose that will have exactly the same degree of effect in all individuals. For some people, one aspirin tablet will cure a headache, whereas it may take two or even three tablets to be effective for other people. Further, consider the differences among people in their tolerance (or lack thereof) to alcohol.

Individual susceptibility to chemicals occurs in all species. That is why acute lethal doses are expressed as averages or means rather than as absolute values. For example, 10 mg/kg of parathion will not kill every rat to which it is administered. It will kill approximately half of a group of rats, but the remaining half will require a larger dose for a lethal effect. Among the half that died, most would have succumbed to a lesser dose.

It is known that some differences among individuals with regard to their susceptibilities to the toxic effects of chemicals are based on differences in genetic makeup (genome). There are a number of well-defined and documented genetic traits that render their possessors more susceptible than the general population to the adverse effects of chemicals and physical agents. For example, people who have red blood cells that are more fragile than normal due to a certain enzyme deficiency are more susceptible to chemicals that cause hemolysis. People who have a genetic deficiency of a certain DNA-repair process suffer from xeroderma pigmentosa, a disease that renders them tremendously more susceptible to the carcinogenic effects of ultraviolet radiation on the skin. Albinos, and fair-skinned people in general, are more sensitive to the damaging effects of sunlight.

Anyone interested in the subject of genetic variations in susceptibility to specific chemicals and physical agents will find the book by Edward J. Calabrese (Suggested Reading section) most useful and informative. Roger J. Williams, who is generally credited with the recognition and development of the concept of biochemical individuality, has also written extensively on the subject. Dr. Williams' books, a few of which are listed in the Suggested

Reading section, are not only instructive but are also very enjoyable reading for a lay audience.

Genetic variations in susceptibility to chemicals are often called genetic defects, which is a misnomer for cases in which the variation is protective rather than damaging. For example, people who have a lowered ability to produce the enzyme AHH (aryl hydrocarbon hydroxylase) are not able to hydroxylate polycyclic aromatic hydrocarbons such as benzpyrene. Since scientific data indicate that benzpyrene must be hydroxylated in order to become the potent carcinogen that it is known to be, the inability to produce AHH is protective. The lack of ability to produce AHH may be responsible, at least in part, for the fact that not all people who are heavy smokers of long duration develop lung cancer. The lack of AHH could be protective against the carcinogenic effects of the polycyclic aromatic hydrocarbons in tobacco smoke.

The fact that there is still a great deal more to be learned about individual reactions to chemicals is exemplified by people who have hypersusceptibilities that cannot be explained by current knowledge. Some of these cases are so implausible that the victims tend to be dismissed as eccentrics. But in my own experience, the people who have contacted me to discuss their extreme hypersusceptibilities to a variety of environmental chemicals all have been intelligent, often highly educated, and reasonable people who obviously were not given to hysterics. Fortunately, severe hypersusceptibilities are rare, but for the individuals so afflicted, their illnesses are personally very tragic.

For some, the problem may be allergic in nature, but for others there appears to be no answer at the present time. However, there is a ray of hope. The recent and exciting advances in the understanding of immunologic tolerances and intolerances to biochemicals within one's own body and to foreign chemicals are convincing evidence that ultimately the solution to many cases of hypersusceptibility will come from the science of immunology. An excellent article, "The Wars Within," explaining the immune system in lay terms, was written by Peter Jaret for *National Geographic* (**169**(6):702–734, June 1986). A more detailed discussion of the science of immunology can be found in the book *In Self-Defense* by Steven B. Mizel and Peter Jaret (see the Suggested Reading section).

PRESENCE OF OTHER CHEMICALS

The toxicity of chemicals can also be modified by the presence of other chemicals. In some cases, the toxicity may be increased (synergism); in others it may be decreased (antagonism). When chemicals act synergistically, the toxic effect observed is greater than would be predicted from data for the individual chemicals; that is, the effects are more than simply additive.

Synergism might be likened to 2 plus 2 equaling 5 (or any other number greater than 4). When chemicals act antagonistically, the toxic effect of the combination is less than what would be predicted from the individual toxicities. Antagonism might be likened to 2 plus 2 equaling 3 or less.

The best understood, and perhaps the most important, mechanism whereby chemicals synergize or antagonize one another is interference in the metabolism of one chemical by the other. Thus, synergism and antagonism may be likened to two sides of a coin. If metabolism converts a chemical to a more toxic form, inhibition of metabolism by another chemical will prevent that conversion and the toxic effect will be less than predicted (antagonism). If metabolism converts a chemical to a less toxic breakdown product, inhibition of metabolism by another chemical will prevent detoxification and the resulting toxic effect will be greater than predicted (synergism). If a chemical increases rather than inhibits the metabolism of another chemical, the above results would be reversed. The chemical would increase (synergize) the toxic effects of a chemical converted to a more toxic form and decrease (antagonize) the effects of a chemical converted to a less toxic form.

There are considerable data in the scientific literature on synergism and antagonism of acute effects between individual chemicals and classes of chemicals, but almost nothing relating to chronic effects. An exception is the well-established fact that smoking synergizes the carcinogenic properties of asbestos. Based on studies of asbestos workers, the risk of lung cancer in a smoker exposed to asbestos is twenty to thirty times greater than a nonsmoker exposed to the same asbestos concentrations.

The lack of information about chronic synergistic effects is not because chronic interactions do not occur or that they are not important but rather because the study of such interactions is so very difficult and so very costly, both in time and money. Hopefully, the chapter describing methods (Chapter 12) will help clarify why this is so. The problems involved with the chronic toxicity testing of individual chemicals are greatly compounded when consideration of synergism and antagonism by other chemicals is added to the protocol. There are so many thousands of chemicals, both natural and synthetic, to which some human populations have a significant exposure that just deciding which combinations of chemicals should be tested, and in what order, becomes a herculean task and probably also a very controversial one. However, the difficulties do not dissuade toxicologists from interest in the subject of chronic interactions among chemicals or from attempts to design experimental methods to overcome the difficulties.

ADAPTATION

Adaptation is a term applied to the process whereby exposure to subtoxic doses of a chemical renders a person tolerant to subsequent doses of the chemical in quantities that would be harmful to nonadapted individuals. Probably the most dramatic example of mass adaptation is that of the fabled arsenic eaters of Styria. People of this mountainous region in central Europe ate small quantities of arsenic trioxide, found naturally in the area, once or twice a week for health purposes. They finally accustomed themselves to doses of as much as 400 mg of arsenic trioxide a day, a quantity that would cause serious illness or death in ordinary people. The arsenic eaters were reputed to have had longer than average life spans.

Adaptation can occur with many chemicals. Two such chemicals most familiar to the general public are alcohol and nicotine. Many people who can handle a three-martini lunch can remember back to the time when a one-martini lunch produced the same glow. And there probably are few smokers who could forget the nausea produced by that first covert cigarette.

The phenomenon of adaptation was referred to as habituation in the early medical literature. It was considered to be due to changes in degree of absorption of the chemical involved. Today, with the increased understanding of biochemical mechanisms, it is recognized that many cases of adaptation are the result of responses by enzymes that process the chemical in question.

The discovery of adaptive enzymes, also known as inducible enzymes, is a fascinating story that has its beginnings in the early research into the metabolic fate of simple nutrients in single-celled organisms. It was long known that if yeast cells were placed in a medium containing glucose, the monosaccharide of table sugar, they started multiplying immediately. It was also observed that if yeast cells were placed in a medium containing galactose, a monosaccharide of milk sugar, they stayed quiescent for a while, then started multiplying slowly, then faster and faster, until they finally achieved the same rate of increase as if they had been placed in glucose solution to begin with. Further, when these yeast cells that had been forced to grow on galactose were harvested and then returned to a medium containing galactose, they did not show the lag time that they had formerly shown, but rather started multiplying immediately. They had the necessary enzymes already available as a result of their prior exposure to galactose.

This behavior on the part of yeast cells, combined with many other similar observations in yeast and other microorganisms, led to the theory that the potential to produce certain enzymes is present in all cells, but that the actual enzymes are not produced until they are needed. Thus, yeast cells placed in a galactose medium do not grow immediately because the enzymes needed to metabolize galactose are not present. But, the ability to produce the enzymes is present, so that when yeast cells are offered galactose as their food source, they slowly form the enzymes required to metabolize galactose. These enzymes are induced by the presence of the chemical they metabolize—their substrate. How very efficient! Why expend the energy required to produce an enzyme if it is not needed, or before it is needed?

Since the discovery of inducible enzymes, it has become recognized that all of us, within the cells of our bodies, contain many inducible enzymes. In fact, some biochemists believe that all enzymes are inducible enzymes, and that those that are always present in our cells are those for which the substrates, such as the common nutrients, are always present. Inducible enzymes explain why we can develop a certain amount of tolerance to a certain number of foreign chemicals. The ability to produce these enzymes, possibly accompanied by trace quantities of the actual enzymes themselves, is present and waiting in our cells for the substrate to come along to be acted upon. As the concentration of substrate increases, so does the quantity of enzyme increase, up to a certain level that is dictated by cellular biochemistry.

The process of adaptation by means of inducible enzymes is not available for all foreign chemicals, nor can it protect a person totally against ever-increasing amounts of toxicant. Even inducible enzymes can be overwhelmed by too much, too often.

LIGHT

Light, artificial or natural, is not considered a factor that influences the toxicity of chemicals. A possible exception is the effect of light on the metabolism of bilirubin in the blood of newborn babies. Bilirubin, a yellow-colored, biochemical waste product, is discharged into the bloodstream when excess red blood cells are destroyed by the body shortly after birth. This is a normal process. However, unless this bilirubin is promptly metabolized and excreted, it can build up in the blood to the point where it causes a serious disease known as neonatal jaundice (hyperbilirubinemia). It was a common disease of the newborn that was difficult to treat. Today, because doctors know that light greatly enhances the metabolism of bilirubin in newborn babies, skin exposure to light is used as a safe and effective treatment for neonatal jaundice.

It has long been known that light exerts a profound influence on physiological responses in animals, including control of reproductive cycles in some species. In the early twentieth century it was discovered that exposure to sunlight could prevent the dreaded bone disease rickets in humans. The role of sunlight in vitamin D synthesis in human skin followed soon after. Scientific interest in the influence of light on human physiology and pathology increased in succeeding decades. As a result, the observation that some people suffered increased periods of depression during fall and winter months led to the recognition of a disease entity now known as seasonal affective disorder (SAD). The symptoms of SAD are fatigue, sadness, excessive sleepiness, craving of sweets, and weight gain. Proof of the role of light is the successful treatment of SAD with light therapy. Exposure to bright light for an additional 5 to 6 hours a day abolishes the symptoms of SAD.

The fact that light is physiologically active in humans and animals justifies its inclusion in this chapter. Photosensitization reactions described in Chapter 2 may be a manifestation of an influence of light on the toxicity of chemicals. Readers interested in the subject will find more information in the New York Academy of Sciences publication edited by Wurtman, Baum, and Potts listed in the Suggested Reading section.

7

ACUTE TOXICITY

Acute toxicity refers to the ability of a substance to do systemic damage as a result of a one-time exposure of relatively short duration. Such exposures are usually accidental in nature. A great deal is known about the acute oral toxicities of a great many chemicals. Experiments designed to determine acute oral toxicity are relatively easy to perform and are not very expensive. The methods of study of acute toxicity are outlined in Chapter 12.

LD_{50}'S AND LC_{50}'S

LD_{50} is the technical term used to describe the acute oral or dermal toxicity of chemicals. LC_{50} is used to describe acute inhalation toxicity. LC_{50} is also used to express the toxicity of chemicals to fish or other aquatic organisms. In aquatic studies, LC refers to lethal concentration of a chemical dissolved in water. LD means lethal dose and is expressed as milligrams of chemical per kilogram of body weight. LC means lethal concentration and its units are milligrams of a chemical per cubic meter of air or per liter of water. When the chemical in air is in gas or vapor form its units may also be expressed as parts of a chemical per million parts of air. The subscript refers to the percentage of the animals for whom the dose was lethal. For example, a subscript of 50 means 50 percent of the animals died, 100 means 100 percent of the animals died, and 0 means no animals died. LD_{50}'s and LC_{50}'s are read from plots such as that shown in Figure 7-1. The smaller the LD_{50}, the greater the toxicity of the chemical, and conversely, the larger the LD_{50}, the lower the toxicity. This inverse relationship between LD_{50} and degree of

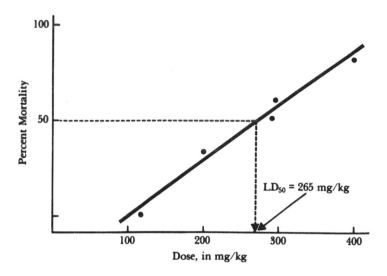

Figure 7–1.   Acute dose–mortality (LD_{50}) curve.

acute toxicity is very confusing unless or until one becomes familiar with the use of LD_{50}'s.

For a variety of reasons, there are many more oral and dermal LD_{50}'s recorded in the scientific literature than there are LC_{50}'s. Many chemicals do not become airborne easily. For these chemicals it is often difficult or impossible to achieve air concentrations that are harmful, much less lethal. For chemicals that do become airborne easily, the technical difficulties of administering known and constant concentrations of gases, vapors, or dusts to groups of animals in environments isolated from laboratory personnel have only been solved in relatively recent years. Most of the knowledge of acute toxicity by inhalation has come from the occupational setting, where people have learned by experience what air concentrations make them feel ill or giddy, or are too irritating to be tolerable.

SIGNIFICANCE OF LD'S FOR HUMANS

The most important source of information about the acute toxicity of chemicals for humans comes not from LD_{50}'s but, unfortunately, from deliberate poisonings and from accidental poisonings. When homicides, suicides, or accidents occur, some estimate of the quantity of chemical to which the victim was exposed usually can be made. That quantity can then be related to the outcome, that is, severity and kind of symptoms, survival, or death. For many chemicals, human experience corroborates animal

Table 7-1.   LD$_{50}$'s and Probable Lethal Doses for Humans

	Lethal Dose	
LD$_{50}$ (mg/kg)	For a 10-kg Child	For a 70-kg Adult
Up to 5	Up to 1 drop	Up to $\frac{1}{16}$ tsp
5-50	1 drop-$\frac{1}{8}$ tsp	$\frac{1}{16}$-$\frac{3}{4}$ tsp
50-500	$\frac{1}{8}$-1 tsp	$\frac{3}{4}$ tsp-3 tbsp
500-5,000	1 tsp-4 tbsp	3-30 tbsp
Over 5,000	Over 4 tbsp	Over 30 tbsp (1 lb)

Equivalents

				0.001	g	=	1 mg	=	1000 μg
		1 drop	=	0.05	g	=	50 mg		
		$\frac{1}{16}$ tsp	=	0.3	g	=	300 mg		
		$\frac{1}{8}$ tsp	=	0.6	g	=	600 mg		
		$\frac{1}{4}$ tsp	=	1.2	g	=	1,200 mg		
		$\frac{1}{2}$ tsp	=	2.4	g	=	2,400 mg		
		1 tsp	=	4.7	g	=	4,700 mg		
		1 tbsp	=	14.2	g	=	14,200 mg		
1 oz	=	2 tbsp	=	28.4	g	=	28,400 mg		
8 oz	=	16 tbsp	=	227.2	g	=	227,200 mg		

toxicity data. If a chemical is shown by data from humans to be more or less toxic to humans than to laboratory animals, human data must take precedence.

LD$_{50}$'s are sometimes used to estimate lethal doses for humans; however, when doing so it must be recognized that they are based on animal experimentation. Reason and judgment must be used to translate their meaning to human terms. When using an oral LD$_{50}$ to estimate the quantity of chemical that would be potentially lethal for a child or adult, the weight of the person (in kg) is multiplied by the the LD$_{50}$ value for that chemical (in mg). A 22-pound child weighs 10 kg; thus, the LD$_{50}$ is multiplied by 10. A 154-pound adult weighs 70 kg, making 70 the multiplier. For example, potentially lethal doses of a chemical with an LD$_{50}$ of 10 mg/kg would be 100 mg for a child and 700 mg for an adult. The relationship between oral LD$_{50}$'s for animals and the quantities of chemical they would represent for children and adults is shown in Table 7-1.

Table 7-1 demonstrates very clearly that children should be protected from acute exposure to all chemicals, regardless of how innocuous they may seem to be for adults. A chemical having a probable lethal dose of about 1 pound for an adult would only require about 4 tablespoons to be lethal to a child; 4 tablespoons is not a very large quantity! Excluding differences in sensitivity to chemicals because of age, lethal doses of chemicals are smaller for children than for adults because children are smaller in body weight. Differences in body weight also account for the fact that insects, with body weights that are minuscule compared to those of humans, are killed by very tiny amounts of insecticides, amounts far below those that are acutely harmful to humans.

It should be mentioned here, if it has not already been made obvious, that the LD_{50} or LC_{50} for humans is not known for any chemical. LD_{50} and LC_{50} values are determined by very specific protocols under controlled laboratory conditions. For obvious reasons, such experiments could not be conducted using humans as experimental animals. Despite the nonexistence of human LD_{50}'s and LC_{50}'s, they nevertheless are given for a number of chemicals in some toxicology reference books. Actually, what these publications really are referring to are not true human LD_{50}'s, but rather average lethal doses (ALD) or mean lethal doses (MLD) calculated from accidental or homicidal deaths.

How are LD_{50} data from animals used to estimate the acute toxicity of chemicals for humans? If there is a great deal of concern about human toxicity from a new chemical because it has a potential for extensive human exposure, routine LD_{50} studies in rats and mice are supplemented with studies performed on additional species such as guinea pigs, dogs, and monkeys in an attempt to determine species variability in response to the chemical. Some chemicals are quantitatively very similar in acute toxicity among species and others vary widely. As a general rule, if a chemical has the same degree of acute toxicity for all species tested, it will probably have a similar toxicity for humans. If data from different species of animals vary widely, an estimate of where people may fit in the scheme is difficult to make from routine animal exposure studies. Further information about how the chemical exerts its toxic action is required. However, regardless of best estimates, it is *always* assumed that humans are more susceptible to the adverse effects of chemicals than the most sensitive species tested until, or unless, there is reliable evidence to the contrary.

The slope of the dose–mortality curve also provides information that is very useful in evaluating potential acute toxicity of chemicals for humans. The slope may be steep (see Figure 7-2A) or it may be shallow (see Figure 7-2B). What is the significance of the slope? Its importance lies in the fact that it provides information about how variable individuals within a species are in their responses to the chemical in question. It tells if the lethal dose range is narrow (steep slope) or wide (shallow slope). If the slope is steep, it means that, within the species, there is only a small difference between the dose that is lethal for the most susceptible animal and the dose that is lethal for the most resistant animal. Conversely, if the slope is shallow, it means that there is a wide difference between the lethal doses. Even though a chemical may show large variations in LD_{50} with species, the slopes of the dose–mortality curves are usually very similar among species, that is, if a

A. Steep Slope

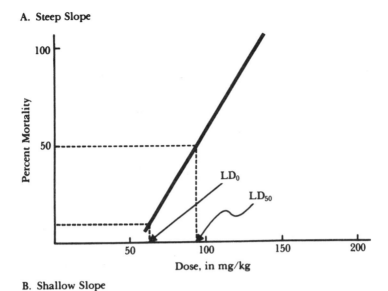

B. Shallow Slope

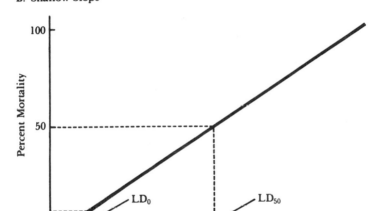

Figure 7-2. Slope of LD_{50} curve.

slope is steep for rats, it probably will also be steep for mice, dogs, monkeys, and so on.

If the slope of the dose–mortality curve is steep, individuals within a species will behave very similarly to each other in their response to the chemical in question. Thus, humans probably will also show little individual variation in the quantity that will produce an adverse effect. The organophosphate pesticides are a group of chemicals that, as a class, have steep dose–mortality curves for laboratory animals. Human experience shows that humans also have little variation in their responses to this group of chemicals. For many organophosphates, doses of up to a quarter or a third of the LD_{50} dose will produce no deaths at all (see Figure 7–2A). A steep dose–mortality slope gives much more assurance than a shallow slope in estimating what a safe acute dose might be for humans. Where human life is involved, the concern is for safe doses (LD_0's) and not doses that will kill 50 percent of the people exposed.

If the slope of the dose–mortality curve is shallow, it indicates that there is considerable variation in susceptibility to that particular chemical within a species. A small fraction of the LD_{50} will be lethal to some individuals (see Figure 7–2B). If test animals show such variation, humans probably would also. In such cases, how an individual human will respond to the chemical cannot be predicted. Therefore, it must be assumed that all humans are as sensitive as the most sensitive person.

An example of a chemical with a shallow slope is diethylene glycol, one of the chemicals used to formulate permanent antifreeze. As little as a tenth of the LD_{50} dose is lethal to some animals. Extrapolation of such data to humans is fraught with danger. An episode involving elixir of sulfanilamide, described below, tragically demonstrated that the slope of the diethylene glycol dose–mortality curve is also shallow for humans.

In 1937, the wonder drug sulfanilamide had just become available for general medical use in the treatment of bacterial infections that before that time had almost always been fatal. One formulation was dispensed as an elixir of 10 percent sulfanilamide, 72 percent diethylene glycol, with the balance being flavoring and coloring substances. Diethylene glycol was selected because it was a good solvent for sulfanilamide. There was little information in the scientific literature at the time relating to the acute toxicity of diethylene glycol. The pharmaceutical company that formulated the drug was unaware of its potential danger. Shortly after the elixir was put on the market, reports began appearing in newspapers around the country about deaths from the new wonder drug. The American Medical Association was deluged with calls from physicians wanting information on the causative agent. Was it the sulfanilamide, the vehicle, or some contaminant? The use of sulfanilamide was totally suspended. Within a short time, diethylene glycol was found from animal studies to be the offending agent. Diethylene glycol was immediately banned as a vehicle for drugs, but not before 100 or more people were made ill and at least 76 people had died from the elixir. Among people who survived, as much as 10 oz of elixir had been taken, whereas among those who died, as little as 1 oz had caused death.

POISON PREVENTION

Fortunately, mass poisonings, such as occurred in the diethylene glycol episode, were uncommon in the past. They are even more unlikely to occur now because of the greatly tightened controls built into food and drug regulations since this episode. Today, the victims in the great majority of cases of acute poisoning from accidental ingestion of chemicals are young children. The tragedy in these statistics is that most, if not all, of these unfortunate events are preventable. After all, how could a child accidentally drink furniture polish if the furniture polish were not made accessible to the child?

Parents may protest that it is not possible to watch toddlers at every moment of the day, especially when there are several young children in the family. This is true in many cases. Therefore, the key is to establish habit patterns of use and storage that keep the many and varied household products, garden products, medicines, and so forth that enter the home environment out of the child's reach. All adults should make themselves aware of the factors that contribute to accidental ingestions among children. They should take steps to make sure these factors do not become operative in their own homes if children live with or visit them.

The most obvious factor is, of course, accessibility. For decades, poison prevention educators have been urging the public to read and heed the labels of all products brought into homes, and to keep every object that is not a toy out of the reach of children. The notable lack of success that this approach has had is attested to by poison prevention legislation enacted in 1970 requiring that certain potentially harmful products be packaged in child-proof containers. Aspirin, which prior to the 1970s accounted for 20 to 25 percent of all deaths from accidental poisoning among children, was one of the first products required to be so packaged. Within a few years after this requirement became effective, the fatality rate from aspirin ingestion by children was reduced by more than half.

Several other factors that play a role in accidental ingestions among children have been identified by the Los Angeles Medical Association Poison Control Center (PCC), which was started in 1957 as the Thomas J. Fleming Memorial Poison Information Center. The work load of the Los Angeles PCC grew from several hundred calls a month in the 1950s to over 4,000 calls a month in the mid-1980s. The records kept on each call provided the center with a great deal of information, including age, sex, product involved, and time of call.

Within 10 years of operation, it became evident to PCC personnel that many of the episodes had certain features in common. One related to age. It had long been known that age was a factor in childhood poisonings, with almost all such cases occurring in children under the age of 5. Data from the Los Angeles PCC refined the age factor. Essentially no accidental ingestions occur in children below the crawling age. The number increases until it peaks between the ages of 2 and 3. After 3 years of age, the number drops rapidly so that by the age of 5, a child is unlikely to become an accidental poisoning statistic. Any parent could explain these data. The child at greatest risk is one who has reached the age of sufficient coordination to find, hold, and pour a container but not the age of sufficient experience and knowledge to understand that all things are not edible.

A second factor, not recognized before its proposal by the Los Angeles PCC, relates to time of day. Poisoning episodes involving children occur primarily during the daylight hours. Within daylight hours there are two peaks, one from 10 A.M. to noon and the other from 4 P.M. to 6 P.M. These are the hours just before lunch and dinner, respectively. Children are hungry and more apt to eat anything they can put their hands on. If the parent is busy preparing food, little attention is being paid to what the child is doing.

A third observation by Los Angeles PCC personnel is that some toddlers are what might be labeled repeat performers, whereas other children, sometimes even in the same family as repeaters, just never become victims of accidental ingestion of chemicals. Repeaters seem to be very active, bright youngsters who are forever getting into some kind of mischief. What actually makes some children accident-prone is not understood, but it could be the subject of an interesting study.

A parent who keeps all nontoys out of the child's reach and is especially alert to what the critical-age-group child is doing at all times, especially during the critical hours before lunch or dinner, is a parent who will probably never suffer the panic of a poisoning emergency. Of greater importance, the child of such a parent will probably never suffer the fright of a trip to an emergency room or the pain and discomfort of a stomach-pump procedure.

Adults can also become victims of accidental intoxication, although the numbers are far fewer than cases involving children. As with children, such accidents are usually the result of carelessness or ignorance on the part of others. Probably the most common cause of accidental poisoning in adults is the storage of pesticide solutions, solvents, household cleaners, or other chemicals in soft drink bottles or other kinds of food containers. Unsuspecting victims drink or eat from containers they believe contain the food specified on the label. Such containers are usually left in easy reach on a table or shelf somewhere in the home. There even have been instances in which containers used for storing excess pesticides or cleaning solutions have been found in refrigerators by unsuspecting victims.

On a much larger scale, accidental spills of chemicals during transportation, either by railroad or truck, and massive accidental releases from industrial processes have the potential for acutely poisoning large numbers of people who have the misfortune to be in the vicinity when the accident occurs. The accidental release of an industrial chemical in an occupational setting can also result in multiple poisonings. However, such releases are often much smaller in scale, and usually affect only one or a few people.

Industry has a responsibility to anticipate likely accidents, take steps to prevent them, and make plans for emergency response in the event that an accident does occur. In addition, people who work with chemicals have a right to know about the toxicity of those chemicals so that they can take proper precautions to protect themselves during normal work procedures.

ANTIDOTES

There is a common misconception in the public mind that when a person has ingested a toxic substance and is rushed to an emergency room, the attending physician administers an antidote which, if given in time, reverses the course of what otherwise would be a fatal outcome. Unfortunately, such is not usually the case. An antidote is a chemical that by one mechanism or another counteracts the action of another chemical, thereby preventing it from exerting its toxic action. Many people believe that for every poison there is an antipoison (antidote). There are actually very few antidotal chemicals. In the great majority of cases of acute poisoning, all a physician can do is to try to remove as much of the toxic material as possible from the victim's system, treat whatever symptoms may be present, and support the life functions of the individual until the body's own restorative powers take over. This course of action, which is usually the only one available to emergency room personnel, is referred to as symptomatic and supportive treatment. Further, the few antidotes that are available may in themselves be toxic. Their administration does not necessarily ensure success. Too vigorous treatment with an antidote also can be lethal.

Some people who are concerned about poisoning by pesticides have demanded that no pesticide be registered unless it has an antidote. This demand is a rather visionary one, albeit a noble and desirable one, because of the paucity of antidotal chemicals. Actually, legislation prohibiting the marketing of any chemical that does not have an antidote would not affect the class of chemicals we call pesticides as adversely as it would other classes of chemicals that we use every day—household products, cosmetics, hobby products, automotive products, paints, varnishes, and so on. This is because, fortuitously, the majority of pesticides actually do have antidotes. A large number of pesticides are organophosphate compounds for which atropine or the chemical known as 2-PAM are antidotal. Many rodenticides are coumarin compounds that exert their toxic action by interfering with blood coagulation. Vitamin K is an antidote for these compounds. Arsenic insecticides have an antidote known as BAL. Acetic acid (the acid in vinegar) and its salts are antidotal for the very highly toxic rodenticide sodium fluoroacetate. Carbamates, another large group of pesticides, have atropine as an antidote. The few remaining commonly known antidotes are listed below.

Chemical	Antidote
Carbamate insecticides	Atropine
Coumarin compounds	Vitamin K
Cyanide	Nitrite, thiosulfate
Fluoride	Calcium
Iodine	Starch
Lead or iron salts	EDTA
Methanol	Ethanol
Nitrite	Methylene blue
Organophosphate insecticides	Atropine, 2-PAM
Oxalate	Calcium
Sodium fluoroacetate	Acetic acid

It is interesting to note that nitrite, which has an antidote for its toxic effects (methylene blue), also can serve as an antidote for another chemical (cyanide).

Fortunately, mild acute intoxications, regardless of chemical involved, almost invariably produce no demonstrable permanent injury. Recovery is complete and health is restored. This is also true for most cases of severe poisoning if the victim responds well during the first critical hours or days after poisoning. The human body has remarkable restorative powers. There are a few notable exceptions, however, such as permanent blindness after severe methanol poisoning and nervous system damage from some of the potent hallucinogenic agents. An attending physician is the most reliable source of information concerning the prognosis for complete recovery in cases of severe acute poisoning.

8

CHRONIC TOXICITY

Chronic toxicity refers to the harmful systemic effects produced by long-term, low-level exposure to chemicals. Far less is known about the chronic toxicity of chemicals than is known about their acute toxicity, not because the subject is of any less importance or interest but because chronic toxicity is much more complex and subtle in its manifestations. Many symptoms of mild chronic intoxication are slow to develop; thus, the connection between exposure and illness may be obscured. In some cases, the symptoms may mimic those of other chronic diseases and, as a result, may be difficult to distinguish from some human ills to which man is naturally prey.

The bulk of information available in the scientific literature on the chronic toxicity of chemicals relates to oral toxicity. The reason for this is twofold: first, some of the earliest concerns about chronic adverse effects were directed toward chemicals used in production, processing, and preservation of foods; thus, it was logical to study their oral toxicity. The second reason, and probably the more compelling one, is that the easiest and most convenient method of exposing test animals to chemicals is by the oral route. It is only in relatively recent years that the importance of the skin and lungs as routes of chronic exposure to chemicals and the importance of using the same route in animal studies as that which is the usual route for human exposure have become recognized.

The methods of study of chronic toxicity are described in Chapter 12. Data obtained from studies of chronic toxicity in animals are plotted on a graph to give a dose–response curve like that shown in Figure 8-1. A dose–response curve has three parts. The first part of the curve is flat. It shows the range of doses that produces no detectable effect. The second segment of the curve begins at a point called the threshold and increases with in-

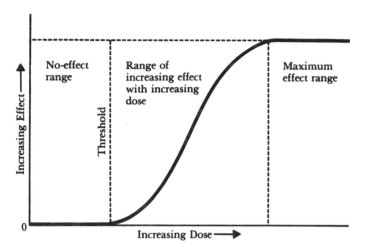

Figure 8-1. Dose–response curve.

creasing dose until the maximum effect occurs. The third part of the curve is again flat, like the first part. Effects described by the dose–response curve may be adverse, such as in toxicity studies, or beneficial (therapeutic), such as in pharmacological studies.

The curve is interpreted as follows: With chronic exposures of doses from zero up to the threshold, no effect is detectable because some biochemical or physiologic mechanism, which may be considered a defense mechanism, handles the chemical in a manner that prevents an effect from occurring. At the threshold, the defense mechanism is saturated, or in some manner overwhelmed, and effects begin to appear. This second part of the dose–response curve, from the threshold to maximum effect, describes a fundamental principle of toxicology: The degree of effect increases with increasing dose. With increasing doses, increasing numbers of animals show the effect until finally a dose is reached where all of the animals show the effect. This third section of the curve is flat because the maximum effect has been achieved; no greater effect can occur with increasing dose.

The same type of curve can be drawn to describe the responses, either chronic or acute, of an individual to increasing doses of a chemical. Below the threshold, no effect is seen. Above the threshold, effects appear, increase in number and severity, and finally a dose is reached that the individual can no longer tolerate and death supervenes.

The dose–response principle, the relationship between dose and effect, aids in the interpretation of data obtained from chronic toxicity testing in animals in the low-, medium-, and high-level exposure groups. If an adverse effect increases with increasing dose, the effect is most probably due to the test chemical. If an effect occurs to the same degree, the effect is probably not due to the test chemical because there is no dose–response relationship. If the effect occurs in the low exposure group and to a lesser extent or not at all in the middle or high exposure groups, the effect is almost certainly not due to the test chemical. In either event, further experimentation may be necessary to clarify the matter.

NO-EFFECT LEVELS AND THRESHOLDS

How are the data obtained from chronic toxicologic investigations used to make judgments about their significance for human health? Unfortunately, there is no nice, neat quantitative expression like the LD_{50} for acute toxicity that can be applied to chronic toxicity. Instead, concepts such as no-effect levels, thresholds, and margins of safety must be relied upon.

The no-effect level of a chemical is an experimentally determined quantity. It is that quantity of chemical to which laboratory animals are chronically exposed, expressed in ppm in the diet or mg per kg of body weight, that produces no effect when compared with control animals. Obviously, the no-effect level in a given experiment will vary with the caliber of scrutiny to which the animals are subjected. The more gross the parameter being measured, the greater the quantity of chemical required to produce a detectable difference between experimental and control animals.

Conversely, the more subtle the parameter being measured, the less the quantity of chemical required to produce the effect. For example, some of the older, classic liver function tests are much less sensitive indicators of liver damage than the newer procedures that measure the activity of certain liver enzymes. A considerable amount of liver damage must occur before it can be detected by liver function tests, whereas liver enzyme patterns can show change with very minimal amounts of damage. Thus, a quantity of liver toxin that would be a no-effect level when measured by the older, classic liver function tests could be an effect level when measured by liver enzyme activity. As a general rule, the no-effect level is taken to be that dosage of chemical to which experimental animals are chronically exposed that produces no harmful effect detectable by toxicologic techniques that are generally accepted by the scientific community as being current and appropriate.

The term *threshold* is used in toxicology to describe the dividing line between no-effect and effect levels of exposure. It may be considered as the maximum quantity of a chemical that produces no effect or the minimum quantity that does produce an effect. The threshold for a given effect can, and usually does, vary with species, with individuals within a species, and perhaps even with time in the same individual. A threshold is, therefore, an elusive quantity that is impossible to determine precisely and directly by experiment. Even if the threshold of an effect in a given individual could be ascertained, it would only apply to that effect and for that individual. Despite the fact that thresholds in individuals cannot be determined precisely, the existence of thresholds is generally accepted as fact. The threshold concept is of great importance to the understanding of the toxic action of chemicals.

It is accepted that thresholds exist because it can be determined experimentally that certain low levels of exposure will produce no detectable effect, and that as the dosage is increased the effect appears. Since the dose-response relationship is a continuum, somewhere between the experimental no-effect and effect levels is the turning point known as the threshold. For purposes of extrapolating animal data to humans, the highest level of exposure that produces no detectable adverse effect of any kind in any of the test animals is used by toxicologists as the threshold.

MARGINS OF SAFETY

The uncertainties inherent in extrapolating data from animals to humans requires that margins of safety be used in the process. A margin of safety is an arbitrarily established separation between the highest level of a chemical that produces no adverse effect in any animal species and the level of exposure estimated to be safe for humans. The FDA adopted the convention of a 100-fold margin of safety many decades ago when it first began setting standards for acceptable quantities of food additives, such as colors and preservatives, that legally could be added to processed foods.

The assumptions behind the 100-fold margin are that (1) humans are 10 times more sensitive to the adverse effects of chemicals than test animals are, and (2) the weak in the human population (young, old, debilitated, etc.) are 10 times more sensitive than healthy adult humans. Multiplying 10 times 10 gives the 100-fold margin. Thus, for example, if the highest level of a chemical that showed no adverse effects in any animal species tested was 100 ppm in the diet, the maximum dietary concentration of that chemical that could be considered safe for humans would be 1 ppm.

This is a much oversimplified example of the kind of calculation that is made in extrapolating data from animal feeding studies to humans. The 100-fold margin of safety is not set in concrete. In fact, it has been facetiously suggested that if man had been created with 8 fingers instead of 10, the classic margin of safety would probably have been set at 64 (8 times 8). Many other factors, such as the toxicities of the chemical by skin absorption and inhalation relative to its toxicity by ingestion, the potential for exposure by routes other than oral, the kinds of foods that will contain the chemical and the relative contribution of each food to the total dietary intake, the need for the use of the chemical, the existence of other less toxic chemicals that could serve the same purpose, evidence of mutagenicity, teratogenicity, or carcinogenicity, and data from human experience with the chemical, are all taken into consideration in the official deliberations and hearings that precede the establishment of standards for chemicals that may legally be added to human or animal foods.

In recent years there has been a demand for regulatory agencies to adopt a 1,000-fold margin of safety, rather than 100-fold, in their standard-setting procedures. Proponents claim that an extra 10-fold margin of safety is required when toxicity data are considered to be insufficient, which is the usual case. Perhaps the 1,000-fold margin of safety is just an inversion of the logic that says if a little is good, more is better—if a little is safe, less is safer.

Actually, there is no more scientific justification for a 1,000-fold margin than there is for a 100-fold margin. If an exposure standard is one that appears to be reasonably protective, reducing it by a factor of 2, 10, or 1,000 cannot make it more safe. The important point is not what margin is used, but rather that all factors related to use of the chemical, described above, are taken into consideration and that a permissible exposure level is set well down in the no-effect range. For some chemicals, a small margin of safety is completely protective, whereas for others a larger margin is required.

The threshold concept and margins of safety are of great importance to toxicologists because they permit them to make judgments about the potential hazard, or lack thereof, to humans from long-term exposure to very small quantities of foreign chemicals. However, they do not permit them to answer questions that are most often asked by public officials, legislators, legislative aides, and regulatory staff people as well as by private citizens. The majority of such questions ask about how large a chronic exposure to a specific chemical can individuals or populations tolerate without any ill effect. It is very difficult, even for people with some scientific knowledge, to accept the fact that no one knows, or can know, what the maximum safe chronic exposure (or the minimum harmful exposure) for all people is for any chemical.

SUFFICIENT CHALLENGE

Although the effects produced by chemicals are usually thought of as being detrimental, this is not necessarily the case. Every toxicologist who has been engaged for any period of time in research into chronic toxic effects of chemicals has observed, more often than not, that animals in the group with the lowest exposure to a test chemical grow more rapidly, have better general appearance and coat quality, have fewer tumors, and live longer than the control animals. More than two decades ago, the late Henry F. Smyth, Jr., a noted toxicologist, proposed the term *sufficient challenge* for this phenomenon in a paper that appeared in *Food and Cosmetics Toxicology* (5:51, 1967). More recently, in a comprehensive work documenting the contradictory effects (detrimental and beneficial) of a host of physical and chemical agents, Walter A. Heiby applied the more encompassing term *reverse effect* for the phenomenon (*The Reverse Effect,* p. 55. Deerfield, IL: MediScience, 1988).

The phenomenon of beneficial effects from exposures to trace quantities of foreign chemicals, although often a subject of conversation among toxicologists, particularly with regard to why such effects occur, is rarely mentioned in the scientific literature. If the phenomenon does occur in a chronic toxicity experiment, the text of the paper reporting the results will seldom mention the fact. It is only by careful perusal of the data tables and figures presented in the body of the text that the phenomenon is revealed. Such subtleties are lost on people who read only the abstracts of scientific papers. Unfortunately, there are some scientists who may be counted among the abstract-only readers.

The reluctance on the part of toxicologists to acknowledge and discuss freely the observation that trace quantities of foreign chemicals can produce beneficial effects may be founded partly on the fact that they have not, as yet, formulated a unified theory for the phenomenon. Or, it may be due to the reality that we live in a time when it is not politic to make favorable statements about synthetic chemicals. Toxicologists who work for industry are particularly hesitant to discuss the phenomenon publicly. No matter how scrupulous an industry scientist may be in maintaining objectivity in his scientific evaluations and judgments, any statements he makes are rejected by some people as being biased.

Since toxicologists recognize that the phenomenon has little practical significance (unless it could be put to some therapeutic use), they have no compelling reason to emphasize it; they might be misunderstood and, as a result, lose a reputation for objectivity. In the absence of any public benefit, why open oneself to attack from people ready to seize upon any statement that sounds prochemical and be labeled by them as an industry apologist? Dr. Smyth learned firsthand how easy it is to be misunderstood; his first use of the term *sufficient challenge* earned him the epithet, "Dr. Smyth and his fellow poisoners."

Figure 8–2 represents how the concept of sufficient challenge (reverse effect) changes the shape of the dose–response curve. With small doses, no effect on the health of the experimental animals is seen (points a to b). Animals receiving slightly higher doses have better than normal health (points b to c, the range of sufficient challenge or reverse effect). At point

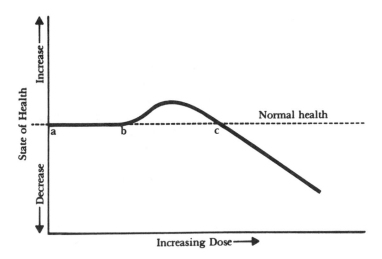

Figure 8-2. A complete dose–response curve.

c, the curve passes back through normal health and, from that point on, deleterious effects occur.

A general acceptance of the concept of sufficient challenge would have no impact on chronic exposure standards or the regulatory procedures that govern them. The prohibitive cost of experimental determination of beneficial effect dose ranges, the impossibility of determining individual responses to such doses, and public concern about environmental contamination all operate against any practical application of the concept. If the public were aware of its existence, it could help to lessen the emotional damage done by an unreasonable fear of chemicals. The concept could also help bring a very necessary public objectivity to the subject of environmental chemicals.

BIOACCUMULATION

No study of the chronic toxic effects of chemicals would be complete without a discussion of bioaccumulation. *Bioaccumulation* is a term that is commonly used, but apparently has different connotations for different people. It is considered by some people to mean the accumulation of cellular or tissue injuries as a result of exposure to chemicals. It is more popularly used to refer to an increase in the concentration of a chemical in specific organs or tissues over that which would normally be expected to be present. This is the meaning that will be used in the following discussion. It should be noted here that storage and bioaccumulation are not synonymous. Storage means deposition of a chemical in some anatomic site. Bioaccumulation is the process by which the quantity of a chemical is increased in an anatomic site.

There is probably no concept in toxicology that is less understood, even in the scientific community, or more frightening than this phenomenon referred to as bioaccumulation. The public became aware of the concept several decades ago when environmental concerns about chlorinated hydrocarbon pesticides, particularly DDT, were being widely publicized. People are still confused and concerned about what bioaccumulation is and what it means for their health and well-being.

A brief description of the nature of the chemical balances that exist in all living organisms is essential for an understanding of bioaccumulation. All living cells possess a certain specific composition, which, within normal limits, remains constant as long as they maintain their customary good health. Despite the fact that this relatively stable composition makes it appear that living organisms are static organizations, nothing could be further from the truth. All living creatures exist in what is known as a state of dynamic equilibrium. *Dynamic* means moving and *equilibrium* refers to the balance, or equalness, that is maintained within living organisms.

A simple illustration of a state of dynamic equilibrium would be a box that contains a specific number of marbles, where every time some new marbles are added to the box, an equal number of old marbles are removed. The total number of marbles in the box remains constant, but the individual marbles present in the box at any one time are not necessarily the same marbles that were in the box at some earlier time or will be in the box at some future time. If the input of marbles increases, the output will also increase by the same number. If there is no delay between the increased input and the increased output, the total number in the box will remain the same. If there is a delay in the output, the total number in the box will increase as the new marbles are added. The magnitude of the increase will be determined by the length of the delay between the increased input and the increased output. A decreased input will have the opposite effect. So it is with living organisms: There is a steady drive toward the achievement of equilibrium—constant change, but little or no net change. Even the bones in our bodies, which people think of as completely inert structures, contain atoms and molecules that are in a constant state of flux.

With the concept of dynamic equilibrium in mind, let us now look at bioaccumulation. Whether or not a chemical accumulates in an organism depends on how fast it is eliminated (metabolized or excreted) relative to how fast it is absorbed into the body. The time between absorption and elimination will be referred to in the following discussion as the residence time of the chemical. Biological half-life is a more common term used to express the length of time a chemical resides in the body. Biological half-life is the time required for the quantity of the chemical to be reduced by half. The length of time required for the concentration of a chemical to come into equilibrium with the exposure concentration after onset of exposure is referred to as the time to equilibrium.

For chemicals with the same rate of absorption, those with longer residence times have a greater potential for bioaccumulation than those with shorter residence times. If the residence time is very short, little or no bioaccumulation will occur (at least not of the chemical, itself; a metabolite may accumulate, but that is an unnecessary complication at this point). Residence time is dependent on such factors as pathway through the body, rate of metabolism or excretion, and the tendency of the chemical either to be held for a period of time in some metabolic pool or storage site (depot), such as fat or bone. The actual concentration that a chemical achieves in a living organism is regulated by the same kinds of forces that drive the organism's internal biochemical environment toward equilibrium.

The storage of foreign chemicals in various depot sites can involve some very complex physiologic processes and equilibrium relationships. Although, for the sake of simplification, the following discussion will consider only the overall equilibrium between absorption, storage, and elimination, it must be remembered that the blood, which serves as the transport medium for chemicals in the body, participates in the process. Blood has its own equilibrium relationships at the sites of entrance, storage, and elimination of chemicals.

The simplest case involving storage of chemicals occurs when the concentration of chemical to which an organism is exposed remains constant over a prolonged period of time and, after entering the body, the chemical is not metabolized. Before the onset of exposure, there are no molecules of the chemical in the body's storage site. When exposure starts, molecules of the chemical begin entering the depot. Some of these molecules also exit the depot but, because of the time delay between entrance and exit, the number entering is greater than the number exiting. The result is that the concentration of chemical in the depot site gradually increases. With continued exposure, the concentration of chemical in the storage depot continues to increase until finally it comes into equilibrium with the exposure concentration.

At this point, the number of molecules leaving the storage site equals the number entering, and the storage concentration remains constant. Molecules of the chemical are moving constantly in and out, but there is no net change—just like the marbles in the box. If the exposure concentration increases, the storage concentration will gradually increase until it comes into a new equilibrium with the higher exposure. If the exposure concentration decreases, the storage concentration will gradually decrease until it comes into a new equilibrium with the lower exposure. If exposure ceases, the stored chemical will gradually be eliminated from the body.

The quantity of chemical that can be stored in any body depot can never exceed that which would be in equilibrium with the exposure. The chemical cannot remain in the storage depot without being replenished continually from the outside. Thus, the popular notion that foreign chemicals stored in a depot become immobilized and permanently fixed in the body, with additional exposures increasing the quantity stored ad infinitum, has no basis in fact. The claim that our bodies can become "walking time bombs" is nonsense.

The quantity of storage and the length of time required to reach an equilibrium state varies from chemical to chemical and depends on the magnitude of the exposure concentration and the nature of the chemical, that is, its physical, chemical, and biologic properties. Many chemicals have no affinity for any storage depot in the body and, thus, do not store. A few have a large propensity for storage and, with high exposures, can build up to high storage concentrations. The remainder display varying degrees of storage between the two extremes. If exposure to a chemical varies continually in concentration and duration, interspersed with periods of no exposure—as is the case with the great majority of our trace exposures to foreign chemicals in the environment—an equilibrium state is never achieved. In such cases, the quantity stored in the body is also continually changing, but would be considerably less than that which would be in equilibrium with the highest exposure level.

The relationship between magnitude of exposure and storage concentration at equilibrium is not known for most chemicals. One exception is the organochlorine pesticide DDT, which has been the subject of a tremendous amount of investigation, including study of its storage and excretion patterns. Before the use of DDT was banned, the U.S. population, on average, received a daily oral exposure of approximately 0.2 ppm DDT in the total diet during the several decades of heavy use of the pesticide. This level in the diet produced an average DDT concentration of 7 ppm in body fat of the American people. The increase in storage concentration relative to exposure concentration at this low level of exposure was approximately 35-fold.

In studies with rats and mice, a diet containing 20 ppm DDT produced a body fat content of 200 ppm, a 10-fold increase. A diet of 200 ppm produced body fat levels of 600 ppm, only a 3-fold increase. Thus, for DDT, the relationship between exposure and storage concentrations is not a linear one. The total quantity of storage increases with increasing exposure, but low levels of exposure produce relatively larger storage levels than do high levels of exposure. From what is known about storage and excretion of foreign chemicals, it appears that DDT can serve as a model for chemicals that store in body fat.

Another piece of misinformation that has been circulated about bioaccumulation is that it puts every one of us at risk of serious or fatal poisoning. It is claimed that chemicals suddenly released from fat depots in the event of a severe weight loss, such as could occur in the case of debilitating illness or starvation, can cause acute poisoning. Poisoning from rapid mobilization of a chemical from fat stores is theoretically possible in laboratory animals under rigidly controlled conditions of exposure and food intake, but is a practical impossibility in the human population.

The question of whether DDT could be released from body fat with sufficient rapidity and in sufficient quantity to produce symptoms of poisoning was of interest to FDA scientists during World War II, when heavy applications of DDT were being made to prevent pandemic outbreaks of certain insect-borne diseases. In the FDA studies, rats were fed 200, 400, or 600 ppm DDT in their diets for sufficient periods to build up high levels of DDT in their body fat, followed by total withdrawal of feed. Rats receiving 600 ppm suffered marked tremors typical of acute DDT intoxication. Rats receiving 200 or 400 ppm DDT suffered increased irritability, but no tremors.

The practical impossibility of such a circumstance occurring in the human population can be demonstrated also using DDT as an example: Assume a worst-case situation of an obese person being 25 percent fat (a normal, well-nourished person is approximately 10 percent fat). A 140-kg (308-lb) obese person would contain 35 kg (77 lb) of fat. The average concentration of DDT in the body fat of Americans during the years of its peak use was 7 ppm. At that concentration, the 35 kg of fat in the obese subject would contain a total of 245 mg DDT. If the obese person had an extremely high exposure to DDT, comparable to rats receiving 20 ppm DDT per day in their feed, he might have a body fat concentration of 200 ppm, for a total quantity of 7,000 mg DDT. Now, let us assume that the obese person stops eating in an effort to lose weight, and manages to lose all 35 kg overnight. He would suddenly release 245 mg DDT or 7,000 mg, depending on which of the above concentrations applied.

How do these quantities relate to acutely toxic doses for humans? It is known from controlled studies in human volunteers that ingestion of 35 mg DDT per kg of body weight per day, for a period of 4 to 5 years, produced no adverse effects, acute or chronic, in any of the subjects. Assuming that ingested DDT can be equated with DDT released from fat stores, 35 mg DDT per kg of body weight would be equivalent to 4,900 mg DDT per day for the obese subject. It is also known from accidents and volunteer experiments that ingestion of somewhere between 50 and 70 mg per kg is less than an acutely toxic dose. For the obese person, that would be equivalent to between 7,000 mg and 9,800 mg of DDT. The hypothetical obese person would contain less total DDT in his entire body than would be required to produce symptoms of acute illness.

Furthermore, anyone who has ever tried to lose weight knows the absolute impossibility of losing so much weight so rapidly. Human volunteers placed on regimens of total starvation can lose only about 0.6 lb of fat in a day (about 0.25 kg). The quantity of DDT released from 0.25 kg fat containing 7 ppm would be less than 2 mg, a quantity that data from human volunteers strongly suggest is a nontoxic chronic dose. People who are concerned about the potential of acute or chronic poisoning from chemicals stored in their body fat are subjecting themselves to the trauma of needless worry.

Bioaccumulation is not inherently good or bad, but in the public mind it is considered, almost universally, to be the latter. In actual fact, whether it is beneficial or detrimental depends on the context in which it is viewed. The ability of an organism to store a chemical in some anatomic depot can actually be beneficial. It functions as a mechanism whereby the organism is protected from the toxic action of the chemical. The chemical does no harm while it resides in a storage site. For example, lead is a very toxic element for animals. It stores in bone where, like DDT in fat, it is in equilibrium with blood levels which, in turn, are in equilibrium with exposure and excretion. Lead isolated in bone does no harm, but lead in nerve tissue causes very serious damage. The removal of lead from blood by bone prevents the blood lead level from becoming sufficiently high to damage nerve tissue. If lead exposure is prolonged or excessive, the bone storage site becomes saturated and can no longer remove lead from blood. In this case blood lead levels can reach levels toxic to nerve tissue.

A storage depot may be considered to have a buffer function during periods of increased exposure. The chemical is deposited in the storage site, where it is prevented from exerting a harmful effect, rather than building up in the blood to a level where it will do damage to a sensitive organ. When exposure decreases, the chemical is mobilized from the depot and eliminated from the body, thereby freeing the site for some future time when exposure may again increase and storage is required to protect against adverse effects somewhere else in the body. When exposure levels are sufficiently high to saturate the depot, there is no more storage space for the chemical and the protective effect of the storage site is abolished.

Probably the only detrimental effect of the ability of the body to isolate chemicals in storage depots is a psychological one. In the absence of knowledge about the phenomenon, the thought that potentially toxic chemicals are residing in one's body can be very distressing.

9

MUTAGENESIS

The word parts in the title of this chapter are derived from Greek and Latin. *Gennan* is the Greek word meaning to produce and *mutare* is the Latin word meaning to change. Medically, mutagenesis is the production of a change in the genetic material of an organism. Mutagens are physical or chemical agents that produce genetic changes (mutations). Mutations are considered to be the initiating events in the development of cancer and in a few classes of birth defects. Therefore, before considering these topics, it is necessary to have some understanding of mutagenesis and the structures affected by mutation.

THE GENETIC CODE

In every living cell, whether it be microorganism, plant, or animal, there is a system of coded messages that tells each cell how to make more cells exactly like itself. This message system, known as the genetic code, is contained in complex structures known as chromosomes. Chromosomes are composed of molecules of deoxyribonucleic acid (DNA) and are located in the nuclei of cells. There are ribonucleic acid molecules (RNA) in the cytoplasm of cells that also participate in the message system. DNA and RNA molecules are composed of subunits called nucleotides. Each nucleotide is composed of three molecules chemically bound together. The three molecules are a purine or pyrimidine base, a pentose sugar, and phosphoric acid. DNA and RNA nucleotides differ from each other only in the pentose sugar they contain; DNA contains deoxyribose and RNA contains ribose. Almost all nucleotides contain one of only two purine or two pyrimidine bases; therefore there are only four principal kinds of DNA or RNA nucleotides.

DNA nucleotides are joined together to form larger units called genes. The genes are considered to be the smallest units that carry a genetic message, one gene for each single characteristic. The genes, in turn, are linked together in long chains that twist around themselves in what is termed a *double helix*. A long double helix strand of DNA is called a chromosome. James Watson and Francis Crick won a Nobel prize in 1962 for their discovery of the helical structure of DNA.

Despite the fact that there are so few kinds of nucleotides, a tremendous number and variety of genes can be formed by linking the nucleotides together in different sequences using different quantities of each nucleotide. Genes also can be linked together in many different sequences to form a wide variety of chromosomes. The nucleotides may be likened to letters of the alphabet, and genes to words formed from the letters. Letters and words can be combined in a great variety of ways to form sentences that can convey an infinite number of meanings. So it is with chromosomes.

All chromosomes occur in pairs. Homologous chromosomes (the two members of a pair of chromosomes) contain the same sequence of analogous genes. The numbers and kinds of chromosome pairs, with their distinctive gene patterns, are referred to as the genome of the organism. The genome is what determines whether an organism is a microorganism, a plant, an animal, what species it is, and what its physical characteristics are within the species. The physical characteristics of an individual can be extensively modified by environmental factors, traumatic accidents, or deliberate intervention, but these modifications are not inherited from parent to child. The only physical features that are inherited are those dictated by the genetic code.

The number of chromosome pairs varies with species, but all members of the same species and all cells of individuals within that species contain the same number. For example, fruit flies contain 8 chromosomes (4 pairs) and humans contain 46 (23 pairs). A chart of the 23 pairs of human chromosomes, accompanied by the known genetic diseases associated with each pair, is presented in an article by Stephen S. Hall describing Dr. Watson's early research and continuing efforts to map the human genome (*Smithsonian* 20(11):40–49, February 1990). Another very informative article about genes, chromosomes, and inheritance that appeared over a decade ago, but is still timely, can be found in the *National Geographic* (Gore, R., and B. Dale, Awesome worlds within a cell. 150(3):355–395, September 1976).

MUTATIONS

A mutation is a change in the genetic code of a cell that results in some change in its message. If the mutated cell is capable of reproducing itself despite the changed message, it will divide into two cells. The two cells formed will be made according to the new instructions. They will carry and reproduce the new code. The two cells and their progeny will all be different in some way from the parent cell, depending on the dictates of the new code. The difference may be so small that the new cells will seem to be exactly like the parent cell in form and function, or the change may be so great that the new cells will be very different in form and function.

Mutations may occur in somatic cells, the body cells of an individual, or they may occur in germ cells, the reproductive cells. Somatic mutations are not inherited by offspring of the parent in which the somatic mutation resides. If the change is small, the somatic cells derived from the mutated cell would probably survive and reproduce. This group of cells would most probably never be discovered because they would be silent and so few compared to the many, many normal cells surrounding them. If the change is a major one, the mutated cell may die before dividing. If it does divide, the daughter cells may eventually die if they are not compatible or competitive with their normal neighbor cells. If they are compatible and competitive, and there are other cells in the vicinity that contain the same mutation, this grouping of cells may grow together to form a tumor. The tumor may be either benign or cancerous. There seems to be agreement among cancer experts that a certain minimum number of cells in close proximity must undergo similar mutation before a tumor can occur. However, theoretically, one mutated cell could conceivably start the process.

A mutation that occurs in a germ cell (sperm or egg) can be inherited. As with somatic cells, a change in a germ cell may be small and compatible with life, or it may be severe and kill the cell. If the cell survives and a new individual is formed from it, all of the cells of the new individual, somatic and germ cells, will contain the change. If the new individual is successful in reproducing, the mutation has the potential for being passed on to all future generations and becoming part of the gene pool of its species. The role of germ cell mutations in reproductive toxicology will be discussed in Chapter 11.

Mutations may be dominant or recessive, a factor that is very important in germ cells. When mature germ cells (sperm or eggs) are formed, each cell receives only one member from each pair of chromosomes. As a result, each germ cell carries one-half the complement of chromosomes that is normal for its species. For humans, germ cells contain 23 chromosomes (one chromosome from each pair). When a sperm and an egg unite, the two homologous chromosomes find each other and form a new pair. A recessive gene on one chromosome of a pair can be overridden by a dominant analogous gene on the companion chromosome. Therefore, a mutated recessive gene will not express itself, but it can be inherited and show itself in some future generation if it comes into combination with a companion gene that is also recessive. A dominant gene overrules a recessive gene and expresses itself immediately. Thus, a mutated dominant gene will overcome a recessive gene, whether the latter is mutated or not.

Some genes are neither dominant nor recessive, but rather show a blending of the two, as demonstrated by the classic experiments of the geneticist Gregor Mendel with four o'clock flowers. White four o'clocks have a pair of genes for white (WW) and red four o'clocks have a pair of genes for red (RR). The germ cells of red flowers contain one R gene. The germ cells of white flowers contain one W gene. When white and red flowers are crossed, their genes combine to yield all pink-flowered plants (RW). Pink color is the result of blending of red and white. When pink-flowered plants are crossed, the red gene from one can combine with either a red gene or a white gene from the other, yielding a red-flowered plant (RR) or a pink one (RW), respectively. In the same manner, the white gene can combine with a red or a white gene from the other, yielding a pink (RW) or a white (WW) plant, respectively. Thus, when pink flowers are crossed, their R and W genes recombine to produce red, pink, and white flowers in a ratio of 1:2:1.

Color in four o'clock flowers is a very simple example of blending when neither gene of a gene pair is dominant. Many physical characteristics are dictated by more than one gene pair. The gene pairs may display dominant-recessive traits or blending, or combinations of the two, which greatly complicates the expression of a trait.

SIGNIFICANCE OF MUTATIONS

Many people have the impression that mutations are always harmful to an organism, but this is not necessarily the case. Some mutations are harmful, but the majority are apparently of no consequence, and a few may even be beneficial. Beneficial mutations may make individuals more disease resistant, better able to obtain food, or in some way better able to cope with a changing environment. As a result, an individual with a mutation may thrive and propagate, while an individual without the mutation may not be able to survive. If individuals of the latter kind are not able to survive long enough to reproduce themselves, their kind will die off. Without mutagenesis, evolution could not have occurred.

It is interesting to speculate about the tremendous diversity of characteristics found in modern man and the role that mutations have played in variations, such as color of skin, eyes, or hair; stature; size and shape of eyes, noses, ears, and lips; and susceptibility and resistance to disease. For many characteristics it is difficult to see how minor mutations could be anything other than neutral. However, mutations relating to skin color, for example, might be classed as harmful or beneficial, depending on the geographic area in which the mutants live. Prehistoric humans apparently evolved in equatorial zones where the sun was very intense. A light-skinned prehistoric human, without benefit of fur or clothing, would not survive very long because of severe sunburns and resulting infections. Dark skin would be protective against intense rays from the sun.

As prehistoric humans moved away from the tropics to colder climates with less intense sun, dark skin would be a disadvantage due to its lesser ability to absorb the ultraviolet rays of the sun; sunlight is required for vitamin D synthesis in the skin. In areas of weak sunshine, dark-skinned people would become ill or die from vitamin D deficiency, whereas light-skinned people would survive and propagate. Modern man has clothing to protect against excessive sunshine and vitamin supplementation of food to protect against vitamin deficiencies. As a result, the influence of skin color on survival in diverse geographic zones is no longer of importance.

An interesting example of a mutation that was beneficial when it occurred many, many generations ago, but is detrimental in modern times, is the sickle-cell trait. In certain Mediterranean areas, swampy marshlands provided perfect breeding grounds for mosquitoes that carried malaria. The disease was endemic, and many of the young died of malaria before reaching adulthood. But a sickle-cell trait protected its carriers against malaria. As a result, people with the trait could survive to adulthood and reproduce. The number of individuals who died from the anemia that resulted from full expression of the trait was less than the number that would have died from malaria. Because sickle-cell is a recessive trait, full expression of the trait occurs only in offspring of parents who both are carriers of the trait and who each contribute a sickle-cell gene to their child.

Sickle-cell anemia is a very debilitating, life-threatening disease that is usually fatal by early adulthood. In modern times, sickle-cell trait is undesirable because it provides no benefit and may cause harm, both psychological and physical. It is no longer needed to protect against malaria, a disease essentially unknown in the United States and treatable when it does occur. The sickle-cell trait is harmful in modern society because people who are carriers of the trait run the risk of having a child with the disease. A child with sickle-cell anemia bears the physical debility and pain while the parents suffer the psychological trauma of seeing their child suffer.

All organisms have biochemical repair mechanisms within them that protect against mutations. In fact, there are several kinds of repair mechanisms, so that if one fails, another can be brought into play. The process is very complex but, in simplest terms, the repair systems read the DNA code. When they find a mistake or a changed message, they correct the message to make it read as it did originally. Individuals vary in the quantity or activity of their mutation-corrector mechanisms. For example, people who have a hereditary deficiency of the mechanism that repairs the damage done to skin-cell DNA by ultraviolet light may suffer from the disease known as xeroderma pigmentosa, a condition that predisposes to skin cancer.

Mutations are not rare events. All of us normally carry within us a great many mutated cells. The causes, nature, and significance of this background incidence of mutations are not well understood and are matters for speculation. Probably a major cause for spontaneous mutations is cosmic radiation and radiation from soil and rocks, both of which are natural and vary with geographic location. Recent publicity about the presence of radon, a naturally occurring radioactive gas, in home and office environments has brought the issue of natural radiation into public focus. EPA has estimated that the air in 10 percent or more of homes contains excessive concentrations of radon. Information about the problem of radon in homes and its solutions can be obtained from the EPA. We can modify slightly our exposure to natural radiation by increasing ventilation in our homes and offices or by changing our places of residence, but we cannot escape it completely.

MUTATION AND CANCER

Interest in how and why mutations occur has been stimulated to a large degree by the evidence that mutation plays an integral role in cancer development. Scientific investigation of mutagenesis produced by radiations predates that of mutagenesis initiated by chemicals by several decades. The development and use of nuclear weapons during World War II greatly increased scientific interest in radiation-induced cancer and the underlying cause, mutagenesis. However, despite the fact that the first cancer attributed to exposure to chemicals was described as long ago as 1775, when Sir Percivall Pott drew attention to exposure to soot as a cause of scrotal cancer in chimney sweeps, there was little interest in chemical mutagenesis until relatively recent years when the fact that some chemicals could cause cancer was rediscovered.

In the early days of investigation of the mechanism whereby chemicals caused cancer, it was natural to look for clues to the wealth of data already available on cancer causation by X-radiation (X-rays). Since it was accepted that X-rays caused cancer by inducing mutations, it seemed logical to assume that chemicals also caused cancer by inducing mutations, and that the mechanisms of both were the same. All of the evidence available for radiation-induced cellular damage indicated that it was an all-or-none (one-hit) phenomenon; whether or not a molecule within a cell was hit was a matter of chance, but if it was hit, it was damaged. An all-or-none mechanism precludes the existence of a threshold, a level of exposure below which no adverse effect will occur.

The use of radiation-induced mutagenesis as a model for chemical mutagenesis is the basis for the current controversy over whether chemical carcinogens have thresholds. If they behave like radiations, they have no thresholds. In this case, they would act as if they were chemical bullets and produce mutations based on chance hits with DNA molecules. If they behave like chemicals, they have thresholds. In this case, they would follow the same anatomic, physiological, and biochemical pathways to reach and mutate DNA molecules as they do to reach any other site where they produce toxic effects.

Before comparing the similarities and the differences between chemical mutagens and X-rays, a brief description of X-rays and their physical and biologic properties is in order. X-rays are produced when a substance is bombarded by high-speed electrons. The X-ray machines that we see in doctors' and dentists' offices and in hospitals accomplish this by using a high voltage in a vacuum tube to accelerate electrons across a short space to a metal target. Some radiations produced by radioactive materials are called gamma rays. X-rays and gamma rays differ from each other only in their source. X-rays and gamma rays are high-energy electromagnetic radiations that do damage by ionizing the medium through which they pass. Ionization is the production of ions, atoms or molecules that have an electrical charge, positive or negative, as a result of having one or more electrons removed from, or put into, their structures. In addition to X-rays and gamma rays, there are other radiations that can cause ionization, such as alpha particles, beta particles, and cosmic rays.

Radioactive chemicals (chemicals that emit ionizing radiations) are complicating factors in any comparison between the behavior of ionizing radiations and chemicals in their pathways through our bodies because they possess properties of both ionizing radiations and chemicals. They can do damage by virtue of their toxicity as well as by their radioactivity. The radiation damage they do is also dependent on their residence time in the body and the energy contained in the radiations they emit.

Radioactive chemicals are also known as radioactive isotopes. Isotopes are atoms of a chemical element that have the same chemical properties but differ slightly from each other in their weights. Isotopes may or may not be radioactive. Those that are radioactive emit ionizing radiations of varying energies, depending on the chemical identity of the isotope. Since a consideration of radioactive chemicals, chemicals that are themselves radiation sources, is not necessary for an examination of why the mechanism of X-ray mutagenesis was adopted for chemicals, they will not be mentioned further in this chapter. Also, the balance of this discussion will use only the terms *X-rays* or *ionizing radiation* because theories of mutation and cancer causation by ionizing radiation were based primarily on studies of the effects of X-rays and gamma rays (gamma rays behave the same as X-rays in their biologic effects).

A necessary assumption in the translation of mutagenic mechanism from X-rays to chemicals is that X-rays and chemicals behave in the same manner in their pathways through our bodies. Is such an assumption valid? Is such an assumption necessary? The fact that both chemicals and X-rays can produce the same end result (mutation) does not require that they do so by the same means. There are innumerable examples, in all phases of our experience, of identical results being achieved by dissimilar methods.

X-rays and chemicals differ markedly from each other in their manner of entry and exit from the body. X-rays are units of electromagnetic energy that pierce biologic systems in a straight line like bullets; hence the term *chemical bullets* for chemical mutagens (carcinogens). They enter a body from any point on the surface, depending on the location of the radiation source relative to the body. If radiations have sufficient energy to penetrate the skin, depending on what that energy level is, they may (1) pass through tissues and organs unchanged and exit the other side; (2) hit a molecule, lose some energy in the process, and continue on either to hit other molecules or to exit in a lowered energy state; or (3) lose all energy in a collision and be totally absorbed. X-rays that pass through an organism without colliding with a biochemical structure lose no energy in the transit and do no damage.

From many studies it is known that X-rays behave as extremely small units of energy, and that the majority do not collide with any intracellular or extracellular molecules. X-rays simply pass through tissue without interacting with it because, at the molecular level, our bodies are mostly empty space. Ionizing radiations must contact and transfer some of their energy to biological material if they are to modify it in some way. The nature of damage that ionizing radiations do to cells depends on how vital the functions of the molecules are that they strike and modify.

X-rays damage living organisms by physically altering any molecules they strike. The energy required to alter molecules comes from the energy in the radiation. After a strike, the energy in the radiation is less by the amount lost in the strike. A major type of molecular alteration is ionization, the event from which this type of radiation takes its name. Ionization inside a living cell can lead to a sequence of reactions that result in damage to cellular components. Ionizing radiations are random in the molecules that they strike. If they strike molecules critical to the health and integrity of a cell, the cell will be injured and may die if it cannot repair the damage. If X-rays strike DNA molecules, mutations may occur and distort the genetic message. The fate of the mutated cell depends on the severity and location of the mutation.

Chemicals are not units of energy but units of matter. They do not strike the surface and travel through biologic systems in bullet-like fashion. Chemicals are substances that enter a body only if they can pass the barrier at the site of exposure, that is, the lungs, skin, or digestive tract. Once transported across one of these barriers, chemicals follow well-defined anatomic, physiologic, and biochemical pathways through the body. In its travels through the body, a chemical meets many barriers, some of which it can pass and some of which it cannot.

There is not the randomness or chance associated with what pathway a chemical will follow or what biochemical materials it will contact on its passage through a human organism that there is with X-rays. The only randomness associated with a chemical in its pathway through the body occurs at the molecular level. The individual molecules of a chemical that cross a barrier do so in an apparently random manner, in what may be likened to a "first come, first served" situation. The total number and the fate of those that cross a barrier is not random, but rather dictated by the biophysics and biochemistry of the organism. Hits or collisions by X-rays with all sorts of extracellular and intracellular molecules and macromolecules, including DNA molecules, occur randomly and by chance.

The chemical bullet theory patterned after the all-or-none theory for X-ray mutagenesis, simply stated, postulates that one molecule of a chemical mutagen, like one unit of ionizing radiation, is capable of hitting a DNA molecule in a cell, thereby causing a mutation. Some chemicals are capable of altering DNA molecules, but they do so by chemical reaction rather than by physical strike. Such chemical reactions may involve oxidation (removal of electrons) of DNA, transfer of a piece of the chemical from itself to DNA, or transfer of a piece of DNA to the chemical. As with mutations produced by radiations, the fate of a mutated cell depends on the severity and location of the mutation.

The answer to the question of whether chemical carcinogens have thresholds is of tremendous importance for public health and the health and well-being of every one of us as individuals. The answer may never be known with absolute certainty, but eventually it will be approached through study of the physiologic and biochemical mechanisms of the actions of chemicals.

10

CARCINOGENESIS

The word *carcinogenesis* is derived from the Greek words *gennan,* meaning to produce, and *karkinos,* meaning crab. The group of malignant diseases called cancer received their name from the Greek word meaning crab because of their crab-like attack on healthy tissue. Thus, carcinogenesis is the creation or production of cancer and carcinogens are physical or chemical agents that cause cancer.

Cancer is one of the most dreaded of all the diseases that afflict the human race. There are many other diseases that are as life-threatening as cancer, and as destructive of the quality of life, but it is a rare person who will not breathe a sigh of relief when told that his illness is one of these other diseases and not cancer.

So it is with chemicals. The public appears to have little concern for chemicals that destroy lung tissue, or nerve tissue, or kidneys, but chemicals suspected of causing cancer are viewed with great apprehension or alarm. As a result, suspected carcinogens are set apart from all other chemicals and made the subject of special laws and regulations.

Regulation of carcinogens is certainly appropriate, but proper respect for all chemical products that one encounters in work or home environments, not just carcinogens, should be encouraged. It would do much to prevent other severe and debilitating occupational diseases among workers and accidental poisonings of children in the home.

WHAT IS CANCER?

What is this disease called cancer that puts us into such panic, and what is known about the chemical causes? Cancers are malignant neoplasms. *Neo-*

plasm, derived from the Greek words meaning "new" and "formation," is the medical term used to designate any new or abnormal growth, such as a tumor. Neoplasms or tumors may be benign or malignant. Medical science knows a great deal more about the prevention and treatment of cancer than it does about its origin and preclinical development. The popular view that cancer is a single disease is not only incorrect but very misleading. There are large groups of malignant diseases, possibly a hundred or more, all with different etiologies and different prognoses, that are grouped together under the umbrella term of *cancer.*

Malignancies are grouped together under the generic designation of cancer because they all have certain characteristics in common. These characteristics are:

> *Cell proliferation:* Cancer cells grow much more rapidly than normal cells from which they were derived.
>
> *Loss of differentiation:* Cancer cells lose some of the features typical of their normal parent cells and become more primitive.
>
> *Metastasis:* Cancer cells invade and destroy adjacent tissues and spread to other more distant organs where they establish secondary cancers. One of the major differences between malignant and benign tumors is that the latter do not metastasize.

There is a controversy in medical science as to whether or not all benign tumors have the potential for becoming malignant. Some benign tumors do show such a propensity, but others appear to remain benign throughout the lives of their hosts. Proponents claim that these so-called benign tumors would eventually become malignant if the host lived sufficiently long. They further point out that some early stages of malignant tumor formation do resemble those of benign growths. Regulatory agencies have simplified the matter by classifying all chemicals that produce any kind of neoplasm, benign or malignant, as carcinogens, thereby eliminating the need to choose from among conflicting opinions in making their regulatory decisions.

There are four basic types of cancers:

1. *Leukemias:* cancers of certain white blood cells and the tissues from which they are derived.
2. *Lymphomas:* cancers of tissues of the lymphatic system, for example, Hodgkin's disease.
3. *Sarcomas:* cancers of connective tissues such as bone and cartilage.
4. *Carcinomas:* cancers of epithelial tissues that form the inside and outside linings of our bodies, for example, skin cancers. Carcinomas are, by far, the most common type of cancer.

Can cancer be inherited? Medical science recognizes that virtually all cancers have heritable and nonheritable forms. In general, cancers that are inherited manifest themselves at a much younger age than usual. If cancer occurs in a person under the age of 30, and there is no obvious etiologic factor that could be responsible, the chances are good that the cancer is due to heredity. There is also considerable evidence that certain types of cancers, such as breast cancer, tend to run in families. However, it is difficult in many of these cases to rule out the influence of environmental factors.

The mechanism by which cancers cause death is not well understood. Cancers, themselves, are not believed to be the actual killers; they do not appear to release any toxic substances into the body. Instead, it is believed that cancers usually cause death by nourishing themselves at the expense of other tissues and organs of the body, thereby causing the latter to become malnourished and subject to failure. The most common immediate causes of cancer deaths are infections, respiratory failure, hemorrhage, liver or kidney failure, and heart failure.

CAUSES OF CANCER

What are the causes of cancer? For many years it has been recognized that there are geographic differences in the incidence of various types of cancers. It has also been known that when people migrate from one part of the world to another, within a few generations their offspring exhibit cancer incidences typical of their adopted land rather than those of the land of their origin. For example, in Japan, cancer of the stomach is much more common than cancer of the colon, whereas in the United States the reverse is true. Japanese-Americans have a stomach/colon cancer incidence ratio similar to that of their fellow Americans rather than that of their parents.

The hypothesis that geographic differences in cancer incidence are due to environmental factors was first enunciated by Dr. John Higginson in the early 1950s. Dr. Higginson's hypothesis was based on an extensive study of cancer among African black populations as compared with black populations in other parts of the world. He concluded that 80 to 90 percent of all cancers were caused by environmental factors. With the growing concern about environmental contamination during the 1960s, it was only a matter of time before the term *environmental factors* became transformed into *environmental chemicals*. By the mid-1970s, statements to the effect that the majority of human cancers could be attributed to carcinogenic chemicals in the environment became commonplace.

An excellent article by Thomas H. Maugh II reported an interview with Dr. John Higginson (Research news: Cancer and the environment: Higginson speaks out, *Science* **205:**51, 1979) in which Dr. Higginson explained that his conclusions have been misinterpreted "not among the majority of scientists with whom I have contact, but by the chemical carcinogen people and especially by the occupational people." Dr. Higginson further stated in the interview that he views life-style as playing a much more important role than environmental chemicals in cancer causation. Dr. Higginson has estimated that approximately 65 to 70 percent of all cancers are due to life-style, including tobacco and alcohol. Two other components of life-style are diet and behavior. An example of effect of diet is the association of colon cancer with lack of dietary fiber. An example of effect of behavior is the association of cancer of the uterine cervix with early onset of sexual activity.

Dr. Higginson said that, in addition to the 65 to 70 percent of cancers caused by diet and life-style, he considers sunlight to be responsible for approximately 10 percent, occupation 2 to 6 percent, radiation 1 percent, congenital factors 2 percent, medical treatment 1 percent, and the remaining 10 to 15 percent due to unknown causes. Perhaps viruses are included in the unknown cause category.

A number of years ago, the hypothesis that a major fraction of cancers had viral origins was popular. Great hope was held that eventually vaccines would be developed to immunize people against cancer. The viral theory has regained some popularity in recent years. There is a large and growing body of scientific evidence indicating that viruses are involved in the development of certain kinds of cancer, but no anticancer vaccine has yet been developed.

The role of background radiation (cosmic rays, radon, etc.) in cancer causation may well be greater than is generally supposed. It may be responsible for much of what is considered the background incidence of cancer—cancer from unknown causes. A visit to a science museum where devices that detect cosmic rays are exhibited reveals that we are constantly being bombarded with those tremendously high-energy radiations. Theoretically, only one hit out of the billions that shoot through each of us is required to initiate a cancer process. In any event, the background incidence of cancer is sufficient to make meaningful epidemiological studies of agents that are suspected of causing very small increases in cancer incidence, such as proposed for trace exposures to synthetic chemicals, extremely difficult, if not impossible.

The belief that the majority of cancers are due to environmental chemicals is still held by some groups. They say that theories such as Dr. Higginson's remove the blame for cancer from where it belongs, the petrochemical industry, and place it on the shoulders of the victims of cancer themselves. This opinion is summarized in "Blaming the Victim" by Samuel Epstein, M.D. (*The Politics of Cancer,* p. 425. New York: Anchor Press, 1979): "Simply stated, the argument is, 'Modern working conditions are so safe that if a worker gets hurt or sick it must be his or her fault and not the fault of the industry.' The culprit is either the worker's bad habits, such as smoking, or the worker's genetic susceptibility to effects which any normal person would shrug off.''

Independent of where the blame belongs, the people at greatest risk of developing cancer from exposure to chemical carcinogens are people who are exposed to the highest concentrations of these agents. The greatest and most varied exposures to chemicals of all kinds usually occur in occupational settings. But, unfortunately, much more public attention is given to trace environmental pollutants suspected of being carcinogens than to occupational chemicals known to be carcinogenic. Certainly, pollution of air, water, and soil by industrial chemicals should not be sanctioned. However, the fact remains that geographic cancer patterns cannot be explained by urban pollution with low concentrations of synthetic organic chemicals. On the other hand, there are distinct patterns of cancer incidence associated with exposure to chemicals among workers in certain occupational groups.

THE ROLE OF MUTATION

The current theory that mutation sets the stage for cancer development is based on the fact that many chemicals and physical agents that are carcinogenic are also mutagenic. There is general agreement in the scientific community that some, and perhaps even most, cancers do result from mutagenic events. There is also evidence that direct mutation is not the only mechanism. Some carcinogens, such as certain hormones, are difficult to fit into a simple mutagenic mechanism. Also, there is not a perfect correlation between carcinogenicity of chemicals and their mutagenic activity in standard testing procedures.

The discovery that there are genes in human tumor cell chromosomes that are related to the production of tumors in mice has stimulated an important new avenue of cancer research. Previously, certain viral genes, known as oncogenes, had been shown to produce cancers in rodents. These data gave rise to a theory that there may be one or a few oncogenes in every human cell that are the genes that must be mutated if a cell is to be induced to become cancerous. Oncogenes play a role in controlling the growth of cells. Further research has demonstrated that, in addition to oncogenes, there are tumor suppressor genes involved in the cancer process. Research indicates that activation of oncogenes and inactivation (or loss) of tumor suppressor genes are critical molecular steps in transformation of a normal cell into a neoplastic one. These events can occur via mutation.

INCIDENCE OF CANCER

The incidence of cancer is dose-related: The greater the dose of chemical carcinogen, the greater the number of individuals that will develop the cancer specific for the chemical. This is an extremely important point to remember when considering the carcinogenicity of environmental chemicals. Almost all chemicals that occur as trace contaminants in the environment have come from some manufacturing or industrial process. Therefore, there must have been occupational exposures to these chemicals. Occupational exposures to chemicals, because of the very nature of the settings in which they occur and the quantities of chemicals involved, are tremendously greater than environmental exposures. If long experience with a chemical in occupational settings gives no evidence that the chemical is a carcinogen, it is extremely unlikely that exposure to trace quantities in the environment could cause cancer. If it did, the incidence would be so low that it would not be detected; it could not be separated out from the background incidence.

What is the incidence of cancer? Approximately one out of every four people in the United States will develop some form of cancer during his or her lifetime. An incidence of 25 percent is a compelling reason for every one of us to learn more about this group of diseases, their causes and their prevention. It has been estimated that, with early diagnosis and treatment, the cure rate for all cancers is about 50 percent. Some forms of cancers, such as skin cancer, have a much higher cure rate, whereas other forms, such as lung cancer, have a much lower cure rate.

Of all deaths in the United States, about 18 percent are attributed to cancer (heart disease and stroke account for about half of all deaths). The total incidence of cancer and the prevalence of the various types of cancer vary with geographic location, economic status, and cultural practices. The United States has among the lowest cancer rates in its white population and among the highest cancer rates in its nonwhite population when compared with all other countries, excluding the USSR and Asia for which data are not available.

The incidence of cancer in the United States is increasing, decreasing, or staying about the same, depending on which authority one accepts. The statistics provided by the National Institutes of Health (NIH) show that the incidence of the majority of cancers has remained about the same or has declined over the past several decades, with the major exception being lung cancer, which is showing a great and rapid rise in number of cases, particularly among women.

Some scientists insist that a different statistical approach to data on cancer incidence supports their contention that the increased production of synthetic organic chemicals over the past 45 years has been accompanied, after an appropriate lag time (induction period), by a gradual increase in total cancer incidence. Other scientists maintain that such a statistical approach does not tell the true story about cancer incidence. They support the conclusion that there is no cancer epidemic in the United States. The public, however, should accept no one else's interpretation. Instead it should read the publications of the American Cancer Society and the reports of NIH on cancer rates, risks, distribution, and so forth as part of their general education on the subject of cancer (see the Suggested Reading section).

CATEGORIES AND CHARACTERISTICS OF CARCINOGENS

The study of chemical carcinogenesis is complicated by the fact that carcinogens are so very varied in their interactions with living organisms. There is no systematized classification of chemical carcinogens. The designations used in the following paragraphs are used for convenience in describing the various types of interactions. Other authors may use different labels for the same interactions.

Chemical carcinogens may act as primary (direct) carcinogens, procarcinogens (indirect carcinogens), cocarcinogens, promoters, or secondary carcinogens. Primary carcinogens are chemicals that directly initiate a cancer process. They do not have to be converted to another chemical in the body before they are able to react chemically with DNA molecules and cause mutations. Radiomimetic chemicals, chemicals that mimic ionizing radiations in their biological effects, are examples of primary carcinogens. Many of the anticancer drugs that are used, alone or with radiation, in the treatment of cancer are examples of primary carcinogens. It may seem ironic that chemicals that can kill cancer cells can also cause cancer. There is good biological reason for the apparent contradiction: Cells that are in the process of dividing (duplicating their chromosomes) are more susceptible to mutagenic agents than quiescent cells. Since cancer cells undergo division so much more frequently than normal cells, they are much more subject to lethal mutations than normal cells. Primary carcinogens are few in number compared to the total number of chemical carcinogens.

Procarcinogens are chemicals that are not themselves carcinogens, but may be converted metabolically to carcinogens. There are a host of natural and synthetic chemicals that fall into the procarcinogen category, the most widely occurring of which is probably benzpyrene, a product of the combustion of organic matter. Foods that are burned or charcoal-broiled are common sources of exposure by the general public to benzpyrene. The major difference between primary carcinogens and procarcinogens is the requirement for biologic activation of the latter.

Some procarcinogens are not converted directly to carcinogens, but must must undergo several metabolic steps. Other procarcinogens may have two or more pathways of metabolism open to them, one that does not produce a carcinogen and another that does. Vinyl chloride, which is known to be carcinogenic for humans, is an example of the latter type. Experimental data indicate that when vinyl chloride is present in the body in very small amounts it is metabolized to vinyl alcohol by the same enzyme system that metabolizes ethyl alcohol. When the quantity of vinyl chloride exceeds the amount that the enzyme system can handle, another enzyme system comes into play and the vinyl chloride is converted to vinyl epoxide, which is the carcinogenic form. Interestingly, people who drink alcoholic beverages appear to be more sensitive to the carcinogenic effects of vinyl chloride. This may be due in part to the fact that the alcohol is saturating the first enzyme system so that the vinyl chloride goes immediately to the second system, which converts it to the carcinogenic form. Since the majority of chemical carcinogens are procarcinogens, a distinction between primary carcinogens and procarcinogens will not be made here, but both will be referred to merely as carcinogens.

Cocarcinogens are not themselves carcinogens, nor are they metabolically converted to carcinogens; instead, they enhance in some manner the carcinogenic activity of other chemicals that are carcinogens. The recognition that there is a distinction between carcinogens and cocarcinogens is a relatively recent development in the field of chemical carcinogenicity and one that has not yet been fully explored. Much of the early data on chemical carcinogenicity did not differentiate carcinogenic from cocarcinogenic effects. Recent investigations indicate that there probably are quite a few natural and synthetic chemicals that fall into the cocarcinogen category.

When animal tests indicate that a chemical is a carcinogen, further evaluation of the data is required. If a chemical causes a greater incidence of cancer in experimental animals than occurs in controls, but the incidence does not increase with dose, or if the cancers occur in a wide variety of sites, the chemical is probably not a carcinogen, but rather a cocarcinogen that is only enhancing the carcinogenic capability of a variety of natural factors or of carcinogens adventitiously present in the diet, bedding, or general environment of the animals.

There are several different mechanisms that could explain the enhancement by cocarcinogens of the carcinogenic potency of other chemicals. Such mechanisms include increasing the rate of conversion of procarcinogens to their carcinogenic forms, altering their biochemical pathways, increasing the rate of cell division, and interfering with repair mechanisms that undo damage done by carcinogens. Caffeine can act as a cocarcinogen by interfering with DNA repair mechanisms. Dioxin is considered to be a cocarcinogen rather than a carcinogen. The mechanism by which it acts may be by increasing the rate of conversion of procarcinogens. Cocarcinogens may very well be of greater importance in cancer causation in humans than carcinogens themselves.

Promoters may form a separate category, or they may be just a special class of cocarcinogen. They are chemicals that stimulate the growth of cells that have already been mutated by other agents. Some, such as croton oil, appear to play only this function, and do not exhibit any other form of cocarcinogenic activity. Bile acids also seem to function only as promoters for colon cancer. Other chemicals, such a phenobarbital, DDT, and other chlorinated hydrocarbon compounds, may act as promoters in some situations and as cocarcinogens in others.

Secondary carcinogens do not fit into any of the above categories, and are not even considered to be carcinogens by some scientists. Secondary carcinogens set in motion a sequence of events that ultimately lead to some sort of tissue damage. The damage, which is not specific to the chemical, is considered to be the primary cause of the cancer, and the chemical is the secondary cause. Oxalic acid is an example of a secondary carcinogen. Chronic oral exposure to relatively low levels of oxalic acid, such as might occur with large daily intakes of foods containing high concentrations of the chemical, may result in bladder stones. The bladder stones in turn can irritate the lining of the urinary bladder. This irritation can eventually lead to chronic damage, which in turn can lead to bladder cancer.

A number of years ago, in an effort to explain differences between direct and indirect actions, chemical carcinogens were divided into two major categories, genotoxic and epigenetic chemicals. Chemicals that damage genetic material (DNA) and cause mutations directly, such as chemicals that are radiomimetic, were classed as genotoxic. Chemicals that were not themselves capable of damaging genetic material were classed as epigenetic. The original distinction between genotoxic and epigenetic chemicals was used primarily to distinguish between primary carcinogens and procarcinogens. However, the fact that procarcinogens could be converted metabolically to chemicals that can react chemically with DNA molecules has blurred the distinction. Many procarcinogens are now classed as genotoxic chemicals. The epigenetic category is reserved for chemicals that cause cancer by some mechanism other than mutation.

Some chemicals cause cancer in only one or a few species, in only one sex, or in only individuals with certain physical or genetic conditions. There are very few, if any, chemicals that are universal carcinogens, chemicals that cause cancer in all groups of individuals regardless of species, sex, age, and so on. Many carcinogens are capable of causing cancer only by one or two routes of exposure, and not by others. Sugar, for example, when injected under the skin of certain species of rodents, can cause a malignant tumor at the site of injection. Fortunately for people who have a sweet tooth, sugar has not been shown to be carcinogenic by ingestion in any species.

Chemical carcinogens are quite specific in the sites that they attack, usually producing malignancies in only one or a few sites. For example, aromatic amine compounds, such as the aniline dyes, cause urinary bladder cancer; mold toxins, such as aflatoxin, cause liver cancers; certain nitrosamines cause esophageal cancer; and thiourea causes thyroid cancer. Despite the fact of species difference in site of attack, when a chemical is labeled as a cancer causer, the public should ask what type of cancer and what increase in spontaneous incidence of that cancer does the chemical cause.

There is also evidence that deficiencies of certain chemicals can cause or predispose to cancer formation. In this category are chemicals that, in some manner, prevent or retard the aging process in cells. Cellular aging is recognized as an important factor in carcinogenesis. Thus, chemicals that retard cell aging in some manner may protect against cancer, and their lack may enhance aging and carcinogenesis. Vitamin C, vitamin E, beta-carotene, and selenium are chemicals that have been investigated for their anticancer properties. Obviously, it is meaningless to say that a chemical causes cancer by virtue of its absence, but the concept of deficiency states playing a role in the carcinogenic process underscores the tremendous complexity of chemical carcinogenesis.

INDUCTION PERIODS

One of the difficulties in studying the causes of cancer and the carcinogenicity of chemicals is that cancers have relatively long induction times. Induction period, or latent period, is the time between the initiation of a cancer by the carcinogenic agent and the clinical appearance of premalignant or malignant symptomatology. The molecular events that occur during the induction period are not understood. Obviously, exposure to a carcinogen can set in motion a process that remains obscure for a period of time until, finally, clinical symptoms appear. A diagnosis of cancer may not even be made until long after cessation of exposure.

The length of the induction period for a given carcinogenic agent varies with dose: The greater the dose, the shorter the time between exposure and recognition of the disease and, conversely, the smaller the dose, the longer the induction period. When exposure to a carcinogen is repeated, day after day for many years, which is the usual case with occupational exposures, the latent period is obscured: Was the cancer initiated on day 1 of exposure, or after many years? It probably *never* occurs on day 1, except perhaps in the rare case of a single overwhelming dose.

Data from experiments in which animals were exposed to carcinogens for different lengths of time, removed from exposure, and then followed for the balance of their lives show that a preinduction period precedes the induction period. The total length of preinduction plus induction periods decreases with increasing exposure and, conversely, is longer with lower exposure levels. If an animal is removed from exposure during the preinduction period, it will *not* develop cancer. The fact that preinduction periods exist is an extremely important point to consider when evaluating the potential for a brief, one-time exposure to a suspected carcinogen to cause cancers in humans. People who are accidentally exposed to low levels of chemicals suspected of being carcinogens, such as occurs so frequently with PCBs (see Chapter 13) released during transformer accidents, are justified in assuming that they are not doomed by the episode.

Information on lengths of induction periods for exposure to some occupational carcinogens can be obtained from retrospective studies of workers in their postretirement years. The most reliable method for determining preinduction and induction periods is by controlled studies in laboratory animals in which exposure to known quantities of carcinogens is followed by long observation periods during which no exposure to the carcinogens occurs.

ADDITIVE EFFECTS OF CARCINOGENS

The proposition that doses of chemical carcinogens are additive is a very frightening one to many people. In simple terms, additive means that exposure to a finite quantity of one or more chemical carcinogens will result in cancer. It is independent of whether the quantity was taken all at once or divided into smaller portions and taken over a long period of time. To illustrate the additive effect, if 10 doses of 10 mg/kg each produced liver tumors in laboratory animals, the carcinogenic dose would be calculated to be 100 mg/kg. Humans exposed to carcinogens each day in quantities equivalent to 1 mg/kg would reach this calculated carcinogenic dose in 100 days. If the daily human intake was only 0.01 mg/kg, it would require about 27 years to reach the critical dose of 100 mg/kg.

The concept that doses of chemical carcinogens are additive conjures up an image of minuscule quantities of carcinogens being stored away somewhere in a receptacle in the body. When the receptacle overflows or when a critical mass accumulates, suddenly a cancer erupts! All foreign chemicals, whether they are carcinogens or not, follow the same natural laws as those discussed in the section on bioaccumulation in Chapter 8. No chemical has some little apartment in the body where it hides and accumulates for the rest of the life of its landlord. Conceivably, if each small dose did some irreparable damage before it was eliminated from the body, such as might occur with chemicals that damage DNA (genotoxic chemicals), succeeding small doses could each in turn add to the damage that finally could result in clinical disease. Such is the case with chronic toxic effects of chemicals. However, with toxic effects, as with carcinogenic effects, some degree of repair between insults is possible.

The concept that doses of carcinogens are merely additive is much too simplistic and not supported by results obtained in studies of carcinogenic effect of chemicals. Examination of data from numerous chemical carcinogenicity studies demonstrates that such an additive effect may appear to occur over certain small ranges of dose and time. But if all of the total doses administered in entire experiments are calculated, it will be seen that very much larger total doses of chemical carcinogens can be administered without ill effect when given in small amounts over a long period of time than when given in larger amounts over a shorter period of time.

Another facet of additive effect attributed to chemical carcinogens is the ability to act in concert, that is, that 100 molecules of 100 different kinds of carcinogens have the same carcinogenic effect as 100 molecules all of one kind. There has been little scientific investigation in this area, but it is reasonable to assume that different carcinogens that cause cancer in the same site by the same mechanism would act in an additive manner, just as different chemicals that produce the same toxic effect act in an additive manner. However, it is important to remember that chemical carcinogens do not just cause cancer; they cause specific cancers. Further, cancer is not a single disease—there are many different kinds of cancers. Carcinogens may cause cancers in different sites in different species and by different routes of exposure, but within a species, by the same route, they are site-specific. There are no data to support the contention that a chemical that causes cancer in one site would act in an additive manner with chemicals that cause cancer in a different site.

THRESHOLDS

There is no controversy about the existence of threshold doses for chronic toxic effects, but there is a segment of the scientific community that denies the existence of thresholds for chemical carcinogens. The rejection of the threshold principle for chemical carcinogens has its origin in the use of ionizing radiation as the model for chemical carcinogenesis (see Chapter 9). With the passage of time, the simple one-hit model has been expanded into a multistage model, primarily because much data obtained from research

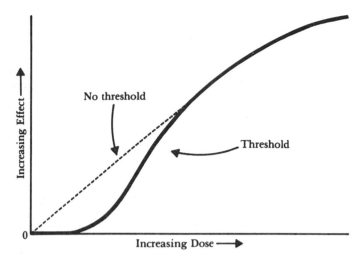

Figure 10-1. Extrapolation of the dose–response curve to zero dose.

on chemical carcinogenesis did not fit a simple one-hit theory. However, thresholds for chemical carcinogens continue to be rejected because their existence cannot be demonstrated experimentally.

Current rejection of the concept of thresholds for carcinogens is rooted primarily in the fact that the shape of the dose–response curve extrapolated from the lowest experimentally determined point down to zero dose is not known. It cannot be known because methodology does not yet exist to describe the curve with absolute certainty. It may go through the origin or it may reach zero effect at some finite dose (see Figure 10-1). If there is no threshold, extension of the experimentally derived dose–response curve to zero effect would yield a line that would go through the origin (zero dose). If there is a threshold, the extended line would meet the abscissa at some point greater than zero dose.

In 1971, the National Center for Toxicological Research (NCTR) was created to provide federal regulatory agencies, such as FDA and EPA, with the scientific data required by them for the performance of their regulatory duties. One of the first missions of NCTR was to shed some light on the question of thresholds for carcinogens. To this end, in 1972 they designed an animal carcinogenicity feeding study of hitherto unimagined size—a "Megamouse" study. The purpose was to answer the question of whether they could accurately describe an ED_{001} for a known carcinogen whose effects had been extensively investigated and were relatively well understood. ED means effective dose (in this case the effect is cancer), and 001 means an effect for 0.1 percent (one per thousand) of the animals in the study.

Such a study, it was hoped, would provide experimentally derived points lower down on the dose–response curve than had ever been obtained before, and, in doing so, shed some light on the threshold question. The physical resources of NCTR, however, could not accommodate the number of animals required by an ED_{001} study. Thus, the plans were scaled down to an ED_{01} study (effective dose for 1 percent of the animals in the study).

The carcinogen selected for the study was 2-acetylaminofluorene (AAF), a chemical for which a great deal of carcinogenicity data were already available. AAF fit the criteria established by NCTR for the test chemical better than any other known carcinogen. The study required 18 months for the planning stage, 9 months for production of the more than 24,000 mice employed in the study, another 3 to 4 years for conduct of the study and evaluation of the data, and cost somewhere between $6 and $7 million. The results of this heroic effort were published in a special issue of the *Journal of Environmental Pathology and Toxicology* (3(3):1–250, 1980).

Evaluation of the massive quantities of data produced by the ED_{01} study required years of effort after the completion of the experimental phase. The study has produced a great deal of information that is of extreme importance to the design and conduct of future studies of the carcinogenicity of chemicals. It will contribute immensely to the development of appropriate models and formulae for carcinogenic risk assessment. However, the question of whether or not a threshold exists for the carcinogenic effects of AAF was not answered. Thus, the question of whether there are thresholds for carcinogens still remains, and may always remain, unanswered. It may be a question that is in the realm of trans-science (see Chapter 16).

Federal regulatory agencies adopted the no-threshold theory of carcinogenesis many years ago when faced with the requirement to make regulatory decisions about chemicals classed as carcinogens, proven or suspected. Their policy was based on the assumption that since radiation "strikes" in biological materials were stochastic (random) events, chemical carcinogen "strikes" were also stochastic events. In stating its policy that the latter was its accepted position, EPA wrote

As defined by the International Commission on Radiological Protection (1977), "*stochastic effects* are those for which the probability of an effect occurring, rather than its severity, is regarded as a function of the dose without threshold." For such effects, which may be regarded as "all-or-none" phenomena, thresholds of "no-effect" levels cannot be established because even extremely small doses must be assumed to elicit a finite increase in the incidence of the response. Carcinogens, mutagens, and, in some cases, teratogens elicit stochastic effects. Consequently, "safe levels"—i.e., levels which will produce no adverse effects—cannot be established for carcinogens and mutagens. (*Federal Register* **44**(52):15,975, March 15, 1979)

PRACTICAL THRESHOLDS

Regardless of the debate over whether there are thresholds for chemical carcinogens, the public should be aware that there are practical thresholds for all carcinogens. There is no disagreement in the scientific community that the incidence of carcinogenic effects and the lengths of their induction periods are dose-related. The greater the environmental exposure to a carcinogen, the greater the number of people in whom it will cause cancer. Conversely the lower the exposure, the smaller the number of people affected. Therefore, if exposure to a carcinogen is sufficiently small as to reduce its cancer incidence to one in a trillion, that level of exposure would be of no practical significance for humans because there are not that many in the world. The chances of getting cancer from that carcinogen would be infinitesimal.

The induction period for cancer, on the other hand, is inversely related to dose. The larger the dose the shorter the induction period, and the smaller the dose the longer the induction period. If the level of exposure to a chemical carcinogen is sufficiently low as to increase its induction period to 200 years, of what practical significance would that be for the human population? The human race has not yet achieved an average life span of 100 years, much less 200.

THE REAL WORLD

Benzpyrene

All humans are exposed throughout their lifetimes to countless numbers of chemical carcinogens, the majority of which are naturally occurring, yet not all humans, or even most, develop cancer. The quantities to which we are exposed are well in excess of the practical thresholds described above. To illustrate, benzpyrene is a naturally occurring and relatively potent carcinogen that is virtually omnipresent in our environment as a product of the cooking or burning of any organic material. It has been determined that there are 50 μg of benzpyrene in about 2 lb of charcoal-broiled steak. A generous portion of steak would weigh about 1/5th of a kg (7 oz). That portion of steak would contain about 10 μg benzpyrene. Ten μg is a very, very small quantity, as demonstrated by the fact that there are over 28 million μg in 1 oz. However, when one considers how many molecules are contained in 10 μg, that seemingly insignificant quantity takes on really formidable proportions. In 10 μg of benzpyrene there would be 24,000,000,000,000,000 molecules! To give this number a name, there would be about 24 quadrillion molecules of benzpyrene in a portion of charcoal-broiled steak. Readers interested in how the number of molecules was calculated are referred to Appendix C.

We do not all eat charcoal-broiled steak every day, but considering that benzpyrene is so widespread in our environment, it is most reasonable to assume that each of us ingests at least billions of molecules of benzpyrene every day (a billion is only one millionth of a quadrillion). The most common site for cancer caused by ingestion of benzpyrene is the stomach, yet in the United States, stomach cancer is one of the less common cancers, accounting for only approximately 10 to 15 percent of all malignancies. On the other hand, benzpyrene in cigarette smoke may possibly contribute to the increased incidence of lung cancer found among cigarette smokers.

If a simple one-hit or chemical bullet mechanism for chemical carcinogenesis were a reality, and if there were no thresholds for chemical carcinogens, what would be the practical consequences? Benzpyrene is only one of a host of natural and synthetic chemical carcinogens to which we are regularly exposed. Even though these exposures are minuscule in practical terms, they represent billions and billions of molecules. If each molecule of a chemical carcinogen behaved as a unit of ionizing radiation, it is difficult to understand how anyone could escape multiple cancers, much less one cancer.

Cancerphobia

The fear of cancer is probably the greatest fear that people have from exposure to synthetic chemicals. This is especially true for pesticide residues and, to a lesser degree, food additives. It is important for people who are concerned about carcinogenic chemicals to remember that someone has synthesized these chemicals and someone has worked with them, usually long before they became available for contact by the general public. As a rule, people in the occupations have been exposed to much higher concentrations of these chemicals, for longer periods of time, than the average person. There is no chemical that is capable of causing cancer whose carcinogenic properties remain hidden for very long after coming into general use in industry. Even vinyl chloride, which causes a rare form of liver cancer in a small percentage of the population occupationally exposed, did not remain undiscovered as a human carcinogen for very many years. This discovery occurred despite the fact that the total number of cases of liver cancer attributed to vinyl chloride is only about 100, worldwide.

Even though prevention of all occupational disease, including cancer, is the major goal of the occupational health professions, the occupational setting will probably always provide the greatest source of human exposure to potentially dangerous chemicals. If a chemical does not cause cancer in exposed occupational groups, it is highly unlikely that it will cause cancer in the general population.

11

REPRODUCTIVE TOXICITY

The influence of chemicals on reproductive function in both men and women has been the subject of considerable research for many years. However, the goal of this research has been the development of methods to interfere with the function (to develop more effective methods of birth control) rather than to protect it. It is only in recent years that protection of reproductive functions and protection of the developing fetus have become the subject of considerable research effort. This research is long overdue and of very great importance.

In years past, before modern methods of contraception were available to prevent pregnancy and before legal abortions were available in the event of failure, self-induced abortion was a social and medical problem of far greater magnitude than it is today. Some women resorted to naturally occurring abortifacients to terminate unwanted pregnancies. Substances such as tansy oil, turpentine, nutmeg, ergot, pennyroyal, and oil of savin (a very toxic oil extracted from a juniper species) have been used since ancient times to induce abortion, often with fatal results. The abortifacient actions of these substances are unreliable, unpredictable, and unsafe when ingested in quantities sufficient to terminate pregnancy.

As toxicologic sophistication has increased through the decades, so has recognition that exposure to some chemicals can produce undesired effects more subtle than previously imagined. Unfortunately, alterations in the reproductive process may be counted among such subtle effects. An excellent review of female reproductive biology and sexuality, with a brief description of male reproductive function, can be found in *Our Bodies, Ourselves,* written by The Boston Women's Health Book Collective (1973. New York: Simon and Schuster).

An almost infinite number of points in the human reproductive process are vulnerable to interference by physical or chemical agents. The reproductive process encompasses the development of the male and female reproductive systems, the maturation and fulfillment of their functions, and the development and viability of new individuals created by the process. Reproductive toxicology deals with adverse effects caused by chemicals at any point in the total process. Because of the very specific nature and complexity of its purview, reproductive toxicology is rapidly becoming a subspecialty in the field of toxicology.

THE MALE AND FEMALE REPRODUCTIVE SYSTEMS

Prepuberty Systems

Under normal conditions, the sex of a new individual is determined by one pair of chromosomes known as the x,y or sex chromosomes. Female germ cells (ova or eggs) all contain one X chromosome. Male germ cells (sperm), on the other hand, are of two kinds. Half of the sperm contain an X chromosome and the other half contain a Y chromosome. When a sperm and egg unite, a female will result if the sperm contributes an X chromosome to pair with the X chromosome in the egg. A male will result if the sperm contributes a Y chromosome.

Early in the life of a developing embryo, a group of cells is set aside to become the reproductive system of the adult. During embryonic and fetal development, the gonads (ovaries or testes) and accessory sex organs are formed. If the individual is a female, the reproductive system remains within the body and a canal (vagina) to the exterior is formed. If the individual is a male, the system is externalized and the testes descend into the scrotal sac. The migration of the testes into the scrotum is an important step in male sexual development. The testes must be maintained at a temperature several degrees cooler than that in the abdominal cavity for the delicate process of sperm production to occur. A male whose testicles remain undescended until puberty, although sexually normal in all other respects, will be sterile.

At birth, the male gonads contain primitive germ cells (spermatogonia). Through a complex process of division and differentiation, spermatogonia will produce many billions of sperm beginning at puberty and continuing throughout the reproductive life of the adult. The female gonads, on the other hand, contain a finite quota of potential eggs, the number of which is determined before birth. The primitive germ cells in the ovaries (oogonia) undergo the first step of development during fetal life to form primitive eggs (oocytes). Each month, beginning at puberty, one oocyte will develop into a mature egg and be released in a process called ovulation. On occasion, two eggs will be released at the same time. Prior to the use of drugs that promote ovulation in the treatment of infertility, it was rare for more than two eggs to be released during one ovulatory period.

There has been relatively little study of the adverse effects of chemicals on the development of the male and female reproductive systems from conception to birth and the maturation and competence of their functions from birth to puberty. Research in this area has revolved primarily around effects of the internal environment, such as hormonal imbalances, disease states, and physical agents, such as radiation. The impact of temperature on sperm production has long been known. Any factor that increases testicular temperature in mature males, such as tight jeans that hold the testicles too closely to the body and perhaps even prolonged exposure to excessive environmental temperatures, can cause sterility or reduced fertility. Male sterility caused by the disease mumps is considered to be due primarily to elevated scrotal temperatures.

The discovery about 20 years ago that some cases of vaginal cancer in prepubertal girls were due to their exposure in utero to the synthetic hormone diethylstilbestrol (DES) given to their mothers during pregnancy emphasizes the fact that there are many vulnerable steps in the reproductive process prior to puberty.

Adult Systems

Puberty, accompanied by production of sperm in the male and the onset of menses and egg production in the female, marks the beginning of human reproductive life. Until recent years, the preponderance of research on the human reproductive process has been directed toward the female with the goal of developing and perfecting more effective methods of birth control. Efforts to develop male contraceptives have increased in recent years. The search for contraceptives has added greatly to the knowledge of female and male reproductive biology.

After puberty, there are many more steps in the reproductive process that can be hindered or impaired by physical or chemical agents. The male must be able to produce good-quality sperm of proper size, shape, and motility. He must produce them in sufficient quantity to be fertile—an average of many millions a day. He must be able to produce adequate transport fluids for the sperm and be capable of delivering them into the female. The male reproductive process terminates when the sperm leaves the body. The only further damage that can be done to the male process is destruction of sperm by contraceptive spermatocides.

The adult female must be able to produce a good-quality egg and release it from the ovary. The egg must be swept into a fallopian tube, the viaduct that delivers the egg to the uterus. The fallopian tubes are where fertilization usually takes place if sperm are present. The egg must be able to permit penetration of a sperm cell for fertilization to occur. If the egg is not fertilized, it passes out of the body and the monthly ovulatory cycle begins anew.

If the egg is fertilized, it must be maintained as it travels down the fallopian tube to the uterus. The first few cell divisions occur during this time. Once the fertilized egg reaches the uterus, approximately a week after conception, it must be able to implant itself in the uterine wall and form a connection with the maternal blood supply so that it may continue to be nourished and grow. The uterine wall must be receptive to the little group of cells destined to become a new individual. The female role in the reproductive process continues through birth and weaning of the infant.

Considerable data are available in the scientific literature that demonstrate the sensitivity of oocytes to destruction by X-rays. Until recent years, the study of the effects of chemicals on oocytes has centered mainly on polycyclic aromatic hydrocarbons, some of which are capable of destroying oocytes in laboratory animals. One such chemical capable of destroying oocytes is benzpyrene, a product of burning organic matter widely distributed in nature. However, there was only narrow scientific interest in the subject of effects of chemicals on male and female germ cells before the discovery in 1977, and the accompanying national publicity, that the pesticide dibromochloropropane (DBCP) was capable of making men who were occupationally exposed to it sterile.

THE DEVELOPING INDIVIDUAL

A fertilized egg that is destined to become a human infant reaches the uterus and implants in the uterine wall approximately one week after conception. At this time it is a little ball composed of cells that are actively dividing. When the little ball of cells implants in the uterine wall, it officially becomes an embryo. It is referred to as an embryo until the end of the eighth week of life. From the beginning of the ninth week until birth it is called a fetus.

After implantation, the embryo forms a sac (amniotic sac) around itself that becomes filled with the fluid in which the fetus will "float" until birth. The embryo and maternal organism then work together to establish a communication system between them. This communication system consists of the umbilical cord and the placenta. The communication system becomes functional around the third week of life. Prior to that time the embryo had to rely on diffusion of products from the uterus (uterine milk) for nourishment.

The placenta forms an intimate contact with the wall of the uterus. The area of contact between the two is called the placental barrier. Blood cells do not cross the barrier; thus, maternal blood and fetal blood do not intermingle. Nutrients pass through the barrier from the mother's blood to fetal blood and waste products pass in the opposite direction. The placental barrier has different permeabilities for different chemicals. Foreign chemicals vary in their ability to cross the barrier. Even some biochemicals, such as the mother's hormones, do not cross to the fetus, at least not in sufficient quantities to interfere with fetal development.

The human embryo, like all other vertebrate embryos, develops from head to tail. The primitive brain, spinal cord, and heart are among the first identifiable structures to appear. By 8 weeks, the head is formed, with eyes, nose, and mouth mapped out, and the upper torso has primitive arms, hands, and fingers. The lower torso is still forming and only little buds indicate where legs will eventually develop. By 12 weeks, the fetus has taken on a more human appearance. All organ systems have been formed and have begun to function. From this time until birth the fetus devotes itself to growth and refinement of physical features and organ functions.

During the 9 months of uterine life there are innumerable developmental steps that are subject to interference or disruption. Congenital malformations (anomalies, abnormalities), more commonly referred to as birth defects, may result from such an interruption. The normal incidence of congenital malformations from all causes in the United States is estimated to be about 2 in 100 live births, and probably about 10 in 100 if mental deficiency is included. Approximately 20 percent of all pregnancies do not go to term, but result in spontaneous abortion. The incidence of fetal abnormalities in this group is not known. Despite such wastage, the fragility of the reproductive process from conception to birth makes the fact that so many newborn infants are born whole and healthy a wonder to many developmental biologists.

There are a host of factors that may cause birth defects, such as disease or malnutrition of the mother, genetic abnormalities, or exposure of the embryo or fetus to physical or chemical agents. Some congenital malformations are so severe that they result in fetuses that are grossly deformed and nonviable. Others that are compatible with extrauterine life run the gamut from mild to severe. A defect may be readily detectable at birth or it may not become manifest until several or many years after birth. When an infant is born with a birth defect, it is often very difficult or impossible to determine what factor was responsible.

One of the major causes of human congenital abnormalities is disease of the mother, particularly viral diseases such as rubella (German measles) during the first 3 months of pregnancy. Another important cause is heredity. Inherited abnormalities are traits that exist in the gene pool, perhaps from mutations that occurred very much earlier in the family line, and find expression when individuals carrying the traits come together as parents. Nutrition plays a very important role in the success of a pregnancy: Starvation or deficiencies (or excesses) of certain vitamins or amino acids can interfere with normal fetal development. Maternal age at the time of conception is also related to the incidence of congenital anomalies. A woman's chances of having a malformed baby begin increasing at about age 30 and take a dramatic upswing after the age of 40.

One process whereby some foreign agent, physical or chemical, produces an abnormality in a developing organism during uterine life is called teratogenesis, a word that comes from the Greek words *gennan,* meaning to produce, and *terata,* meaning monsters. Thus, teratogens are agents that give rise to malformed or otherwise abnormal fetuses. Some chemicals and certain physical agents, such as natural and man-made radiation, can behave as teratogens. Chemical teratogens may or may not be mutagens and chemical mutagens are not necessarily teratogens. X-rays, in particular, are both potent mutagens and teratogens. The use of X-rays during pregnancy, once so popular in obstetrical practice to determine position of the fetus, number of infants, and so forth, is now reserved for very special circumstances.

In order for a congenital abnormality to be produced by a teratogenic agent, the agent must physically contact the developing organism. In the case of ionizing radiations, the embryo or fetus would have to be in the pathway of the radiations as they passed through the mother. In the case of viruses or chemicals, they would have to be capable of crossing the placental barrier.

A teratogen must not only be able to contact the developing organism but it must also reach it during a critical phase in the gestation period when organ systems are in the process of being formed. The dividing egg is considered to be protected fairly well against the teratogenic action of chemicals during the week to 10 days from conception to implantation because of the lack of a direct communication system with the mother. The critical stage of organ development for the human is the first 3 months (first trimester) of pregnancy. The kind of abnormality produced depends on what organ system is undergoing most rapid development at the time of exposure to the teratogen. For example, exposure to high doses of vitamin A on the eighth day of gestation in rats results in skeletal malformations, whereas the same doses on the twelfth day result in cleft palate.

There are very few chemicals known to be teratogenic for humans. Among them are certain steroid hormones, vitamin A, vitamin D, some anticancer drugs, and, of course, the infamous drug thalidomide that was used extensively in Europe during the 1960s for relief of the nausea of pregnancy. There are a number of other chemicals that are suspected of being teratogenic, many of which are industrial chemicals or drugs, about which physicians can provide information. The wisest course for any woman who is pregnant, particularly during the first 3 months, is to observe all rules of good nutrition and avoid smoking, alcohol consumption, and excesses of all kinds. If work or hobbies involve use of chemicals, a woman should seek her obstetrician's advice concerning such exposures.

One of the difficulties with such advice is that a woman often does not know she is pregnant until the fourth or sixth week of pregnancy. By that time some important organs have already been mapped out in the embryo. This fact forms the basis for the dilemma involving women's rights and fetal protection. The question of whether women of childbearing age should be excluded from certain jobs involving exposure to industrial chemicals in order to prevent possible harm to an unrecognized embryo has been presented to the Supreme Court for adjudication (*United Auto Workers* v. *Johnson Controls Inc.*, US SupCt, No. 89-1215, petition filed 1/29/90).*

Chemicals can also produce fetal malformations by a number of different mechanisms other than teratogenesis. They may produce mutations in parent germ cells prior to conception, which in turn result in a birth defect. They may interfere with development of the placenta and thus prevent adequate transfer of nutrients from mother to fetus. They may prevent adequate oxygen transfer to the fetus. They may interfere in the growth of organs or organ systems, or the refinement of their structures or functions, resulting in an anatomic, physiologic, or biochemical defect. They may exert a toxic action on the fetus and thereby cause degenerative changes in one or more anatomic, physiologic, or biochemical systems.

The fetotoxic chemical that probably is responsible for more fetal abnormalities than all other chemicals combined is alcohol, even when taken in the small amounts described as social drinking. Chemicals may also produce acute or chronic intoxication in the mother, causing a generalized debility in her and, secondarily, some adverse effect on the developing fetus. The latter situation is probably rare in humans, except in cases of excessive use of alcohol, illicit drugs, and tobacco, but it can be readily achieved in laboratory animals.

A congenital anomaly resulting from the action of a mutagenic agent on a parent germ cell or on an embryonic cell may result in a changed message for some relatively minor structure or function, or the changed message may result in some major defect. Depending on the nature of the change, the mutation may (1) never be expressed during the lifetime of the individual; (2) show itself in some physical deformity or disease state compatible

---

*On March 20, 1991, the Supreme Court "ruled that employers may not bar women of childbearing age from certain jobs because of potential risk to their fetuses." *The Wall Street Journal,* March 21, 1991, p. B1.

with survival to adulthood; (3) result in a deformity or disease that is too great to permit long-term survival so that the individual dies at birth, in infancy, or in early childhood; (4) cause death of the fetus in utero.

For a congenital malformation to be heritable, the message for the defect must be carried in the germ cells of the malformed individual. Thus, the mutation would have had to occur at some time prior to the segregation of the cells destined to become the individual's reproductive cells. That could have been sometime in the distant past, with the defect carried in the germinal line of the ancestors down to the sperm or egg of a parent. The mutation could have occurred in the immediate past by action of a mutagen on a reproductive cell of a parent or early in the life of the fertilized egg, before differentiation of the cells destined to become germ cells. Malformations resulting from mutations of somatic cells of the fetus will not be passed on to progeny. A mutation in a germ cell will only become part of the human gene pool if the individual carrying it is able to survive to adulthood and reproduce.

12

METHODS OF STUDY

The purpose of this chapter is to give the reader an introduction to the kinds of experiments used to study the adverse effects of chemicals, the limitations of the methods and analytical procedures involved, and the meaning of some of the terms used to describe effects or quantities of exposure. It is not intended to serve as a cookbook for the conduct of toxicity tests. It is beyond the scope of this book to provide more than a brief summary of methods of toxicity testing because they are too many and varied. In some cases, they are very ingenious. Details of testing protocols, both animal and nonanimal, can be found in toxicology and pharmacology texts and journals. In the past several decades, regulatory agencies, such as the FDA and EPA, have formalized the testing requirements and experimental protocols for chemicals that come under their regulatory purview. This information can be obtained from the respective agencies or can be found in the past issues of the *Federal Register.*

The key to relevant toxicity testing in animals is the selection of a species that handles the chemical under study in the same manner as humans do with regard to absorption, metabolism, excretion, and so on. Before such a model can be selected, a great deal of study into the physical and biochemical properties of the chemical may have to be undertaken. Since there is no one species that handles all chemicals in the same manner as humans, there is no one animal model that can be used to study the toxicity of all chemicals for humans. The identification and characterization of animal and nonanimal models for research have given rise to a very important new science based on comparative toxicology.

Among the earliest subjects of toxicity testing were slaves who served as tasters for emperors, kings, and other nobles who feared that some unknown enemy might have slipped poison into their food or drink. There were few other uses for experimental animals until the dawn of modern medical science brought the need for development of surgical techniques and study of efficacy of medications. Undoubtedly, the first experimental animals in modern times were stray dogs and cats. As the need for pharmacological research increased, so did the need for large numbers of experimental animals. Rats and mice were ideal subjects. They were prolific and small. Thus, they could be produced in large numbers and, because of their modest space requirements, could be housed inexpensively. The wild mice, rats, and other rodents that were trapped many decades ago and bred in captivity became the ancestors of today's commercially produced laboratory animals, animals of high quality and known lineage.

ANIMAL RIGHTS

No discussion of toxicity testing methods would be complete without reference to the animal rights movement. The great increase in the use of laboratory animals that accompanied the commercial development of synthetic organic chemicals after the end of World War II was followed by increased public concern for the humane treatment of laboratory animals. Apart from their concern for the welfare for the animals in their charge, scientists who used animals in their research long ago recognized that maltreated or sickly animals were poor subjects because they gave unreliable results. In order to avoid such difficulties, scientists and their member societies gradually developed protocols for laboratory animal care. These protocols eventually became incorporated into federal law in 1967 as the Laboratory Animal Welfare Act.

Laws and regulations requiring humane treatment of laboratory animals are not sufficient for people opposed to the use of animals in research. The fact that laboratory animals are unwitting participants in research, combined with the assumption that such research is always cruel and painful, has given rise to a new rights movement—animal rights. The animal rights movement, as with any movement involving social issues, represents philosophies that range from moderate to extreme. Moderate views recognize that advances in medical and allied research are dependent on the use of animals for some procedures. They advocate the development of methods that do not require living creatures and, when no alternatives are available, that experimental animals be treated in the most humane and least painful manner possible. These goals are also goals of science and the scientists who use animals in research.

Groups with extreme views have targeted animal experimentation for extinction. Extremist views in the animal rights movement have led to extremist tactics, such as destruction of laboratories and research records, liberation of laboratory animals, and even threats and attempts against the lives of research scientists and industry personnel. Unfortunately, those who suffer most from these criminal acts are the very animals that the acts are intended to help. Whenever research records are destroyed, the animals who participated did so in vain. Such research must be repeated, requiring the use of more animals.

The liberation of experimental animals is the cruelest act of all. Animals bred for research are not feral animals capable of surviving against all odds in the wild. They do not have the adaptability of their wild counterparts. They suffer greatly during their short period of survival in the wild. Because they have been bred in captivity for so many generations, they have become totally dependent on their keepers. They have lost all survival instincts. They do not know how to find food or safe shelter. They do not know how to protect themselves from harm, and they have no resistance to the diseases common to their wild fellow creatures.

Research using animals is essential to protect the health and well-being of humans. Animal experimentation is conducted, almost without exception, for the prevention or alleviation of human ills and suffering. Toxicologists would prefer to have nonanimal methods available for their research because animal subjects are extremely expensive to buy, maintain, and use. Despite the claims of some animal rights activists, scientists who use animals for research are not sadists who enjoy inflicting pain on their subjects. On the contrary, they have as much concern for the quality of life of their laboratory animals as they do for their own family pets.

There is considerable interest in finding alternative nonanimal methods of study, and numerous investigations of nonanimal methods are in progress. However, the search is fraught with problems. It is very difficult to find a nonanimal substitute for a human tissue or organ, much less the whole organism. Probably more important is the problem of validation. Once a nonanimal method is found that gives promise of being suitable, how do results obtained with it compare to those from animal studies? How do data from nonanimal systems translate to effects in humans? The answers to these questions must be obtained before a new nonanimal method can be substituted for an older, proven animal method. The process of validation requires a great deal of time, effort, and money.

Readers who are interested in nonanimal subjects should familiarize themselves with organizations such as The Johns Hopkins Center for Alternatives to Animal Testing and The Tufts School of Veterinary Medicine Center for Animals and Public Policy.

Despite great activity in the search for alternate methods, there are, at the present time, some kinds of studies for which no alternate methods are available. In fact, it is conceivable that a substitute for the whole animal may never be found for some kinds of research that are dependent on the interplay of the tremendous number of complex physiological and biochemical processes and interactions in the living organism.

EXPERIMENTAL METHODS

The chemicals on which routine toxicity testing is done are all new chemicals coming into general commercial use. These include such chemicals as pesticides, drugs, food additives, industrial chemicals, and household products. In addition, any older chemicals, in any category, that have come under suspicion since their commercial introduction of causing cancer or any other adverse health effect are subjected to retesting. Since the major concern of people is the carcinogenicity of chemicals, it should be pointed out that only a small fraction of the many thousands of chemicals that have been subjected to toxicity testing or retesting, as a result of regulation by EPA, have been found to be carcinogenic in animals. Because of the patterns of home use of chemicals, and the increasing federal regulation of the use of cancer-causing materials, the percentage of potentially carcinogenic chemicals that find their way into the home setting would be an even smaller fraction.

Acute Toxicity

The methods used to study the acute toxicity of chemicals are relatively easy to perform and relatively inexpensive. Their purpose is to learn what might happen in case of accidental or deliberate exposure to large amounts of chemicals or products. Probably the majority of accidental acute poisonings occur in children, but adults also can be exposed to acutely harmful amounts of chemicals in home or work situations. The general public is at particular risk when chemicals are released in large quantities during transportation accidents.

The classic test for the study of acute toxicity is known as the LD_{50} test. LD means lethal dose and the subscript 50 refers to the 50 percent of the test animals for which the test chemical is lethal. This test is the most commonly performed acute toxicity test. It is estimated to consume many hundreds of thousands of animals yearly, worldwide. There is probably no synthetic chemical available for commercial or home use that has not been subjected to an LD_{50} study.

The classic LD_{50} experiment, described below, is no longer required by FDA for chemicals they regulate; however, data about acute toxicity are still required. In the absence of acceptable nonanimal methods, the only alternative is to design studies that use fewer animals. This was the approach taken by EPA in 1988. In a revised policy on acute toxicity testing, EPA offered several methods that would reduce the number of animals used without compromising public safety. Details of their revised policy may be found in the September 22, 1988, issue of the *Federal Register*.

The test animals for classic LD_{50} experiments are usually rats and mice. Preliminary studies are conducted in order to obtain a general idea of whether the chemical or product is of high, moderate, or low acute toxicity. This information is then used to decide what doses should be administered in the LD_{50} test. The test animals are divided into four or five dosage groups of several animals each. Each animal in the lowest dosage group is administered an amount of the substance that preliminary tests indicate will cause no deaths. Each animal in the highest group is given a quantity of the substance calculated to be lethal to all of the animals. The other groups are given quantities intermediate between the two extremes. The animals are observed closely for a 14-day period. All adverse reactions and deaths are recorded during the observation period. Then the data are plotted on a graph, using statistical methods that convert curved lines into straight lines, to yield what is known as the dose–mortality curve. The quantity of chemical that falls on the point of the curve corresponding to 50 percent mortality is the value taken for the LD_{50} (see Figure 7-1).

LD_{50}'s can be determined for oral and dermal routes of exposure. For an oral toxicity test, the chemical is administered by stomach tube. The quantity of chemical administered is expressed as mg or g/kg of body weight. Chemicals with oral LD_{50}'s of 50 mg/kg or less are classed as highly toxic (poison). Chemicals with oral LD_{50}'s of 50 to 500 mg/kg are considered to be moderately toxic. The toxic range extends up to 5 g/kg. Chemicals with oral LD_{50}'s greater than 5 g/kg are legally classed as outside the orally toxic range, or nontoxic by default. Since any chemical is capable of causing illness under some set of circumstances, toxicologists prefer to consider the latter group as having relatively low toxicity rather than no toxicity.

Dermal LD_{50}'s are determined by placing a weighed quantity of chemical in continuous contact with an area of bare skin that is approximately 10 percent of the animal's total body surface. The test is conducted on both intact skin and abraded skin. The animals used in dermal toxicity studies are usually rabbits because of their larger size and, hence, their larger areas of skin. The period of continuous contact is 24 hours. As with oral toxicities, dermal LD_{50}'s are expressed as mg or g/kg of body weight. Chemicals with dermal LD_{50}'s below 200 mg/kg are placed in the highly toxic (poison) category. Those with dermal LD_{50}'s between 200 mg/kg and 2 g/kg are classed as toxic. Dermal LD_{50}'s greater than 2 g/kg are legally outside the toxic range.

The measure of acute toxicity by inhalation is termed the LC_{50}, which means lethal concentration for 50 percent of the animals tested. LC_{50}'s are determined by exposing several groups of animals, usually rats or mice, each to a different air concentration of a chemical, for a 1-hour period followed by a 14-day observation period. At the end of the observation period, the data are plotted to give an air concentration–mortality curve similar to that for oral or dermal toxicity. The air concentration that corresponds to 50 percent mortality is taken as the LC_{50}. Chemicals with an LC_{50} of up to 20,000 parts of gas or vapor per million parts (ppm) of air or 200 mg dust per liter of air (mg/l) are classed as toxic by inhalation. Those with LC_{50}'s at or below 200 ppm gas or vapor or 2 mg/l dust are in the highly toxic (poison) category. Chemicals with LC_{50}'s greater than 20,000 ppm gas or vapor or 200 mg/l dust are legally nontoxic.

All of the definitions of acute toxicity by oral, dermal and inhalation routes given above are taken from the federal Hazardous Substances Labeling Act (Public Law 86–613, July 12, 1960). The same definitions are used in laws that apply to pesticides and food additives.

Irritant and Corrosive Effects

Testing for irritant or corrosive properties is standard procedure for substances regulated by various federal agencies. Such testing is important to protect people who contact irritant or corrosive chemicals in their occupations. It is even more important for the protection of members of the general public who bring irritant or corrosive products into their homes, particularly homes with small children. The general public usually has less knowledge about how to protect themselves than workers do.

Oral and dermal LD_{50} studies provide information about irritancy and corrosiveness of chemicals as well as their toxicities. In fact, the majority of corrosive chemicals, such as the drain cleaners found under many kitchen sinks, have LD_{50} values that place them in the poison range. These chemicals are not very highly toxic, but their corrosiveness makes them lethal in very small amounts. They cause death by chemically destroying the tissues they contact.

Many products composed of chemicals that are known to be of relatively low toxicity may not require LD_{50} studies, but some investigation of their irritancy properties must be conducted. Tests that give more rapid results are desirable for these kinds of products. There are many such tests available today—animal, nonanimal, and human.

The classic techniques for studying irritation and corrosiveness to skin and eyes were developed many decades ago. They bear the name of J. H. Draize who was chief of the Skin Toxicity Branch of the FDA at the time the tests were developed. The skin tests follow the dermal LD_{50} protocol, except that the holding period is 3 days rather than 14. The degree of irritation is determined by rating the degree of redness, swelling, and/or blistering according to a standardized score chart. The use of human volunteers as subjects for studies of skin irritant properties of substances whose toxicological properties are quite well understood, such as soaps and detergents, is relatively common and probably the most informative and useful method of study of mild irritants.

There is no area of animal testing that has given rise to more public outcry than the Draize test for ocular reactions. In this test, three groups of albino rabbits are used. In all groups, the test material is dropped into one eye of each rabbit, with the other eye serving as a control. In one group, the treated eye is not washed after instillation of the test material. In the other two groups, the treated eyes are washed after two seconds or four seconds. After 24, 48, and 72 hours, and at 4 and 7 days, the results are rated according to a standardized score chart.

There is probably no industry that has a greater need for tests of irritation or damage to skin and eyes than the cosmetic industry. During the past decade there has been a major effort by this industry, in collaboration with drug and chemical companies, to develop testing techniques that would eliminate the need for live animals. Materials such as tissue cultures, chicken egg membranes, and vegetable protein films show great promise as substitutes for chemicals with severe corrosive effects. However, the research and validation demonstrating that any one (or more) are as predictive of damage as the Draize test are not yet forthcoming. At the present time, there is no substitute for an animal eye to detect chemicals that have only mild to moderate eye irritant effects.

Sensitization and Photosensitization

Probably the most common condition for which people seek medical attention is an allergic reaction to some agent. Allergies are seldom fatal, but they are often distressing and, in extreme cases, debilitating. People are so heterogeneous in their susceptibilities to sensitization that it is a rare chemical that has not caused an allergy in some individual. Thus, the major goal of testing a chemical for sensitizing properties is not whether it can be a sensitizer but rather the strength of its ability to sensitize—the percentage of an exposed population it will affect. Because of product liability, it is understandable that information about the ability of a chemical to cause an allergic reaction is probably as important to the cosmetic industry as information about its irritant or corrosive properties.

Guinea pigs are the animal models used for sensitization studies because they are extremely susceptible to a wide variety of chemical sensitizers. Small quantities of the test chemical are injected within the layers of the skin, at random, over a small area of the back or sides, one injection every other day, until a total of 10 sensitizing injections have been made. After a rest period of two weeks, a challenge injection, smaller in quantity than the sensitizing injections, is administered at a site just below the area of sensitizing injections. Twenty-four hours later, reactions are rated according to a standardized score chart.

Obviously, the ideal animal models for sensitization experiments are humans; however, even studies in humans are not always predictive. Before humans are used, some information must be available about how severe reactions might be. Exposure to severe sensitizers could produce long-term adverse effects or even death in human subjects. The guinea pig test is a valuable tool for screening chemicals for the strength of their sensitizing properties prior to human exposure.

Photosensitization studies are conducted in a manner similar to sensitization studies. Since photosensitization may occur after oral exposure as well as dermal exposure, the test chemical may be administered by mouth, applied to the skin, or both. The subject animals are albino rabbits and the challenge test is exposure to daylight or sunlight.

Chronic Toxicity

The purpose of chronic toxicity experiments is to obtain information about the possible or probable adverse health effects that could result from long-term exposure to relatively small quantities of chemicals. There are two levels of concern about the chronic toxicity of chemicals. One concern is for health effects in a population of young and old, healthy and infirm, men and women, exposed to trace quantities of a wide variety of chemicals in the environment. The other is for health effects in people exposed to chemicals in their occupations. The latter exposures are fewer in number for any one occupation, but the quantities of exposure, while still small, are up to tens of thousands times greater than environmental exposures. The study of the chronic effects of chemicals is a complicated, lengthy, and expensive process.

How is the chronic toxicity of chemicals studied? Experimental protocols for chronic toxicity testing are many and varied. The type of chronic adverse effect being investigated governs the selection of methodology. Such factors as route of exposure (oral, dermal, inhalation), nature of effect (organ damage, mutagenicity, carcinogenicity, birth defects, etc.), and objects of concern (adult, child, developing fetus, etc.) are important determinants of the experimental design.

A wide variety of animal species are used in the study of the chronic toxicity of chemicals, ranging from monkeys and other subhuman primates, to dogs, cats, pigs, and numerous rodent species, down through nonmammalian animals, such as birds, reptiles, amphibians, and fish. The most common test animals for chronic toxicity studies are rats and dogs. Subhuman primates would probably find more common use if it were not for their relatively limited supply and great cost. Certain types of toxicologic experiments utilize microorganisms, tissue cultures, or isolated animal organs. These latter kinds of experiments provide valuable information and direction for further investigation, but with our current state of knowledge they cannot yet replace whole animals in the study of chronic toxic effects of chemicals.

The classic chronic oral toxicity experiment is quite simply (and in the minds of some more academically oriented scientists, quite crudely) an animal feeding study. Before a feeding study is begun, range-finding experiments based on a knowledge of acutely toxic doses of the chemical under investigation are undertaken to determine what daily doses the animals would be able to tolerate for prolonged periods. These range-finding, subacute studies are usually about 90 days in duration. Based on the data obtained from these investigations, three or more feeding levels of the toxicant are selected for the long-term chronic study.

The toxicant is mixed homogeneously with the animal feed to give the desired concentration for each feeding level. The highest level fed to the animals is one calculated to have significant sublethal chronic effects. If the high-dose level kills the animals before the end of the experiment, its value in providing meaningful chronic toxicity data is limited. The lowest level fed to the animals is, ideally, one that will produce no detectable adverse effects. The intermediate levels are those that will produce effects intermediate between the high and low levels. One group serves as a control, an essential part of a chronic study protocol. Control animals are treated in exactly the same manner as the experimental animals, except that the test chemical is not added to their feed. Control animals are essential in long-term studies to assure that any adverse effects that occur during the course of the experiment are, in fact, due to the toxicant and not to some other condition of the experiment.

Relatively large numbers of animals are assigned to each exposure group because chronic toxicity studies are for all practical purposes lifetime studies. Thus, some attrition can be expected, even in control groups. When rats are the experimental animals, at least 25 females and 25 males are assigned to each group. When dogs, swine, or monkeys are used, the groups are made up of a minimum of 4 females and 4 males each. The duration of feeding is 24 to 30 months for rats (lifetime) and 6 months to lifetime for nonrodent animals, depending on the protocol. The animals are started on their respective diets at weaning. They are observed daily for any signs of abnormal health or behavior.

All animals are given a more detailed examination weekly, at which time they are weighed, their feed consumption is measured, and any scheduled clinical tests are performed. During the experiment, various other biochemical and clinical tests may be performed periodically in an attempt to determine if any adverse effects that are sufficiently subtle to escape gross observation may be occurring. At the end of the experiment, all animals are autopsied. At autopsy, they are examined grossly for any signs of tumors or other pathologic change. Selected organs are weighed for evidence of atrophy or hypertrophy, and numerous tissues are preserved for microscopic examination for evidence of histopathology. All data are evaluated statistically to determine if there is a relationship between dose and effect.

Figure 8-1 explains a dose–response curve typical of those plotted from data obtained in chronic toxicity experiments. It is very important to recognize that such a curve is drawn from only several points, one for each exposure group in the experiment. The greater the number of exposure groups, the greater the number of points, and hence, the greater the accuracy of the curve that is drawn. However, without an infinite number of points, the precise shape of the dose–response curve cannot be known.

Classic animal feeding experiments and all of their modifications also can be used to investigate dermal and inhalation toxicity of chemicals by merely altering the route of administration. Exposing animals by the dermal route takes a great deal of technician time, and exposure by the inhalation route requires highly specialized and expensive equipment. Technician time and specialized equipment add greatly to the cost of what are already very expensive procedures.

The EPA estimated over a decade ago that a 2- to 3-year feeding study of chronic toxic effects (excluding carcinogenic effects) in two species, following the standards set forth by their agency, would cost approximately $550,000 per chemical. They estimated that a similar study designed to reveal carcinogenic effects would cost approximately $400,000. If the two studies were combined, the cost would be only $800,000 (Proposed rules, VI. Economic analysis, *Federal Register,* **44**(91):27,346, May 9, 1979). It is estimated that today the cost of a chronic toxicity feeding study is about $1,000,000 and that the time required for the study has increased to 4 to 5 years.

The above estimates would be very much greater if comparable experiments employing dermal and inhalation exposure were included. Further, these figures do not include the expense of all of the many preliminary and range-finding investigations that must precede chronic feeding studies, nor do they include the costs of research into effects on reproduction, mutagenic and teratogenic effects, and biochemical and physiologic properties. Even excluding an allowance for inflation, it is probably not unrealistic to estimate that the price for development of what currently is considered to be adequate chronic toxicity data could approach several millions of dollars per chemical.

Any discussion by science or industry of the great costs of chronic toxicity testing should not be viewed as a tacit argument against such investigations. Rather, it is a statement of why such testing is, for the most part, limited to chemicals that promise to have sufficient commercial value to justify the costs. The high cost of toxicologic evaluation is a fact about which the public is generally unaware, but which exerts considerable influence on decisions that affect their health and well-being.

No matter how much time, effort, and money are put into the study of the chronic adverse effects of chemicals, and no matter how many studies yield negative results, one can never be sure that there is not some subtle effect that is yet to be discovered. Each chronic toxicity experiment adds to the fund of knowledge about long-term effects of chemicals.

As we develop a larger and larger data base of chronic effects of chemicals, nontoxic as well as toxic, and as our knowledge of mechanisms of action of chemicals increases, the need for classic animal feeding studies may diminish. Before that time arrives, other problems, such as the chronic toxicity of chemical combinations, and the significance of synergistic and antagonistic chemical interactions, will have to be dealt with.

Reproductive Toxicity

The original methods for the study of reproductive effects were designed by nutritional scientists in the early 1930s. Methods development was stimulated by numerous observations that maternal malnutrition could exert a profound effect on the fetus and the young in the postnatal period. Nutritional studies were gradually extended to investigation of reproductive effects of excess nutrients or other chemicals added to the maternal diet.

Three basic types of studies were developed to study effects of chemicals on reproduction. The first involved administering the test chemical to a female after pregnancy had been established. This method became a tool for teratologists. In the second method, the test chemical was administered to both males and females prior to mating and continued until the young were weaned. The third method evolved from the second. Instead of terminating administration of the test chemical when the young were weaned, exposure was continued until three or more generations were produced. Both the single-generation (second) method and the multigeneration (third) method are still used by toxicologists. The single-generation study is used as a screening test to provide data for planning a multigeneration study.

It has been a common practice during the past 25 to 30 years for multigeneration tests to be conducted on any new chemical that may find its way into the food supply, either deliberately or inadvertently. In multigeneration studies, feeding groups are set up and examinations are conducted in the same manner as described for chronic toxicity testing. When the animals reach maturity, they are bred and permitted to deliver and wean their young before they are submitted to the autopsy examination. Pups from each litter are selected to become the parents of the next generation, and the remaining pups are autopsied. This process is repeated until three or four generations are produced. This type of experiment provides information about whether chronic exposure to the chemical in question adversely affects the overall reproductive process or produces some condition that does not express itself prior to the second or third generation.

In recent years, many more types of tests have been developed to study the nature and location of effects of chemicals in male and female reproductive processes. Some of these tests involve the use of live animals; others involve the use of animal tissues or cells. The techniques employed come from a variety of disciplines, such as physiology, biochemistry, genetics, and molecular biology.

Mutagenesis

The purpose of mutagenicity testing is to study the ability of chemicals to change the genetic code. A number of different methods are used to investigate mutagenesis. Some involve microscopic examination of the nuclei of cells, such as white blood cells or the cells of other tissues, to see if the chromosomes are abnormal in size, shape, or number. Some mutations involve only a subunit of a chromosome and do not alter the gross appearance of the chromosome on which it resides. At the present time, there is no way that geneticists can determine if genes are mutated by looking at them directly. Such mutations can only be detected indirectly when they express themselves in the mutated organism or its progeny.

Mutagenicity studies utilize a variety of test organisms, such as rats, mice, or other mammals, animal tissues, insects or other lower animal forms, plants, or microorganisms. No one test method can adequately describe mutagenic risk for humans. Thus, it is usual for batteries of tests to be employed when evaluating potential mutagenicity of chemicals for humans.

There is one test that has become commonly used for preliminary screening of chemicals for mutagenicity. That procedure is the Ames test named for Bruce Ames, the scientist who developed the technique. The organism used in the Ames test is *Salmonella typhimurium,* a microorganism that has lost its ability to synthesize the amino acid histidine as a result of mutation from its normal wild type. This mutant requires the presence of histidine in its media for it to survive and multiply. In the Ames test, the mutant organism and the test chemical, plus biochemical activators, are placed in media lacking in histidine. A certain number of the mutants will spontaneously revert (mutate) back to the normal wild state and will be able to grow in the absence of histidine. If the test chemical is capable of causing mutations in the organism, the number of organisms that revert back to the wild type will be greater than the number that spontaneously reverts. The greater the number of reversions, the greater is the potency of the mutagen.

Any chemical that is judged to be a potential human mutagen is a chemical for which human exposure should be carefully monitored or controlled. However, there is much irony in the fact that the test most commonly used to screen chemicals for the property of mutagenicity is a test for a chemical's ability to convert a mutated organism back to its normal state.

Carcinogenesis

Because mutation is considered to be a critical event in cancer causation, screening tests for carcinogenic potential of chemicals use some of the same methods as those used in mutagenicity testing. These screening tests give valuable information about carcinogenic potential. However, the ultimate test must be long-term exposure of test animals to the chemicals in question, such as used in studying chronic toxicity. The reason for this is that some chemicals that do not yield positive results in mutagenicity tests do cause cancer in animals, and, conversely, some chemicals that are mutagens are not carcinogens.

One of the shortcomings of animal carcinogenicity testing is related to the long induction periods and low incidences associated with exposure to small quantities of carcinogens. If there is any exposure of the general public to suspected carcinogens in air, water, or soil, it is usually very small, in parts per billion (ppb) or parts per trillion (ppt) quantities. The use of such small exposure levels in laboratory experiments would require astronomical numbers of animals in order to detect a carcinogenic effect. Since such studies are not feasible, the common practice in animal carcinogenicity testing is to administer large doses, tremendously larger than would be encountered by the general public, in order to increase the potential for demonstrating a carcinogenic effect of the test chemical. Heroic doses, referred to as maximum tolerated doses, are the highest nonlethal doses the animals can tolerate for the duration of the experiment.

The use of heroic doses is accepted by regulatory agencies despite acknowledged pitfalls. The public is generally unaware that such pitfalls exist. The pitfalls derive from the fact that the biochemical fate of very small doses of a chemical is usually not the same as that for large doses. The difference in effect that chemicals display between their acute and chronic toxicities is testimony to the fact. Small doses of a chemical may follow a metabolic pathway that does not convert it to a carcinogen. With increasing doses the pathway becomes saturated and the excess chemical is diverted to a different pathway that does convert it to a carcinogen. Or, small doses of the chemical may be prevented from exerting carcinogenic activity by combination with a biochemical normally present in the body. If the supply of the biochemical is expended by large doses, the excess chemical is then free to exert its carcinogenic effect.

The only chemicals for which effects at high levels would accurately represent low-level effects are those whose biochemical fate is not altered by dose, a very unusual situation. Despite toxicologic and biochemical data to the contrary, there are a few scientists who deny that alterations in metabolism occur with high doses.

Some analogies to the use of high doses, ridiculous though they may seem, may give the reader an idea of the kind of distortions that animal tests utilizing high doses can produce. A team of sports physicians is interested in investigating the adverse effect, if any, on the ankle, knee, and hip joints of athletes who participate in pole-vaulting events. The problem is that it would take hundreds of thousands of pole vaulters, making their jumps every day for a period of many years, to obtain sufficient data that could produce statistically significant results. Since such an experiment is impossible, it is decided that instead of 100,000 people making a 20-foot jump each day for many years, 1,000 people will make a 200-foot jump 10 times a day for 1 year. Since no athlete could vault 200 feet, and since the trip up is of no importance to the experiment, a nearby 200-foot cliff is selected as the jumping-off place.

At another university, a group of aquatic biologists is concerned with a problem that involves the impact of a 4°F rise in water temperature on marine life at the site where cooling water effluent from a nuclear reactor will enter the ocean. There is no aquarium large enough to handle a controlled study of a size sufficient to produce meaningful results on the chronic effect of only a 4°F rise in water temperature. Therefore, it is decided to use an aquarium of normal size and increase the temperature not 4°F but 40 times 4°F, or 160°. Since a 160° rise over background would bring the water temperature to near the boiling point, it is decided to simplify the temperature control system by keeping the aquarium water just at the boiling point.

The above analogies grossly exaggerate an indifference to the obvious biologic limitations of the test organisms by suggesting conditions that are greater than the maximum that could be tolerated. Nevertheless, the fact of indifference is the same as it is in carcinogenicity testing using heroic doses.

Proponents of the use of maximum tolerated doses justify their position by saying that maximum tolerated doses do not artificially induce cancer. They contend that if a chemical causes cancer in very high doses, it will also cause cancer in very low doses. This position denies the fact that changes in metabolic pathways of a chemical can occur with increases in dose.

Knowledge of biochemical mechanisms and data provided by study of metabolism of carcinogens belie its accuracy. The use of maximum tolerated doses in animal carcinogen studies does provide valuable information and certainly should not be deleted from testing protocols. However, acceptance of results from high-dose exposures as the only valid data, with concomitant rejection of data from moderate-dose studies and studies of mechanisms of action, metabolic fate, and so forth represents an attitude that is foreign to objective scientific inquiry and a disservice to the public.

A more moderate approach to carcinogenicity testing is the use of doses comparable to those received during occupational exposure to chemicals. Working populations, as a rule, do not include young children, senior citizens, or people who are ill or debilitated, but their lack of representation in occupational groups is compensated for by the fact that occupational exposures to chemicals are usually several to many thousands of times greater than those encountered by the general public. Occupational exposures are sufficiently high to provide valid data using numbers of animals that reasonably can be accommodated in a toxicologic laboratory.

This approach, which provides a compromise between the extremes of trans-science and heroic dosing, is employed by some research scientists investigating the carcinogenicity of chemicals. The use of exposure levels that reflect those found in occupational settings is most appropriate; a chemical that does not cause cancer in occupationally exposed people is very unlikely to cause cancer in the general public, particularly at dose levels that are thousands of times lower than those found in occupational settings.

UNITS OF TRACE QUANTITIES

The terms *ppm, ppb,* and *ppt* have come into common usage in recent years. Everyone knows that ppm means parts per million, ppb means parts per billion, and ppt means parts per trillion. But, what do they really mean? How much is one unit of some substance in a trillion units of some other substance (ppt)? What is its significance? These questions take on even greater importance when one recognizes that analytical chemists are pushing the limits of detection further and further down in the scale of quantification. We must be prepared for ppq (parts per quadrillion), ppp (parts per pentillion), pph (parts per hexillion), and so forth.

How much is one part per million? One part per million is equal to 1 drop in 14 gallons. A ppb is 1/1,000th of a ppm. Therefore, a ppb is equivalent to 1 drop in 14,000 gallons. A ppt is 1/1,000th of a ppb. Therefore, a ppt is equal to 1 drop in 14,000,000 gallons. Or, as a colleague once remarked, "A very dry martini!"

Other colleagues have offered other analogies. A ppm may be likened to the diameter of one hair being expanded to the diameter of the Holland Tunnel. A ppt is equal to the thickness of a dollar bill in a stack of dollar bills 63,000 miles high. All sorts of similar calculations can be made to dramatize the extremely small quantities that ppm, ppb, and ppt represent.

Even though ppm, ppb, and ppt are extremely minuscule quantities, they still represent billions and billions of molecules, as can be seen from the discussion of benzpyrene (Chapter 10). Recognition of this concept is necessary for an understanding of the difficulties inherent in requiring that the quantity of any chemical contaminant in any medium—air, water, food, soil—be zero. Zero, the absence of even one molecule, cannot be measured. Therefore, zero contamination has no practical meaning for any chemical that has any commercial use at all.

The only chemicals that we can say with reasonable certainty are present in the environment in zero amounts are chemicals that have never existed. For all other chemicals, natural and synthetic, the best that analytical laboratories can do is determine that they are not present in amounts detectable by the most sensitive analytical equipment available. The quantity of a chemical that is below the level of detectability depends on a number of factors, such as the nature of the chemical in question and what medium it is present in. The level of detectability becomes smaller and smaller with improvements in analytical techniques, but it will probably never reach zero.

ANALYTICAL METHODS

The public, in general, has complete faith that concentrations of contaminants reported to be present in environmental samples, wildlife species, food, drinking water, and most especially now in organic or pesticide-free produce are accurate and absolute. People who are not chemists do not appreciate the tremendous technical difficulties of measuring ppb or ppt of any chemical in any medium. Analysis of such extremely small quantities requires elaborate and expensive analytical equipment that is not to be found in many laboratories. Further, any laboratory that is capable of accurately measuring ppb or ppt quantities must be impeccably clean; even ppb contamination of solutions, reagents, laboratory air, or the most minuscule traces on glassware, bench surfaces, or equipment would completely obscure the presence of ppb or ppt in a sample. A contaminated laboratory can only give unreliable results. More often than not, a contaminated laboratory will report the presence of a trace amount of chemical when it is actually not present at all in the sample. On the other hand, concentrations of chemicals in the ppb and, more especially, in the ppt ranges are invisible in many laboratories. They are too small to be detected by some analytic instrumentation and methods.

Some laboratories will report an unqualified zero when an analysis does not detect any of the chemical in question. This is a meaningless report because there is no laboratory that can determine zero (that no molecules of the chemical are present). On the other hand, some laboratories will give a figure like "<0.2 ppm." It gives the impression that some of the chemical is present, perhaps as much as 0.199 ppm, when in actual fact all it really says is that the chemical was not detected, but that if it was present it was in a concentration of less than 0.2 ppm. The majority of laboratories report results in the proper manner, which is to state the quantity found (or zero, if none was detected) followed by the sensitivity of the analytical method— the smallest concentration that is capable of being detected by the analytical procedure.

Another problem with analytical procedures for some of the very complex organic chemicals is whether they really detect what they are designed to detect. Whole groups of chemicals can give the same response in some procedures. Without methods for separating the various components of the group, there is no way of knowing which or what combination of them is present in a sample. This was the problem with the early analyses for DDT in environmental samples. Even today, chemical analysis for trace quantities of chemicals is an extremely difficult and tedious procedure.

The question of the significance of the results of chemical analyses should be of particular concern to people who want and demand pesticide-free foods. Consumers should ask what chemicals are detected by the methods used, how sensitive the methods are, and about the competence of the laboratory employed to test their produce. The health effects of exposure to trace quantities of environmental chemicals are independent of whether those quantities are detected or undetected.

The public, in general, also seems to have the impression that analytical laboratories have much greater capabilities than they do. For example, many people who feel they have been made ill by some food or other material often want to send it to a laboratory to determine the identity of the offending contaminant. They do not realize that laboratories can only analyze for specific chemicals or specific groups of chemicals. Laboratories cannot just look for anything. Therefore, the chemical for which the analysis is to be made must be specified. In light of the fact that there are hundreds, if not thousands, of potential contaminants, an analysis of a sample for an unspecified chemical would be a major and extremely costly research project.

Some final thoughts about laboratory analyses: If a physician suspects acute or chronic poisoning from some chemical, such as lead or arsenic, clinical laboratories can provide very valuable and necessary information to assist in the diagnosis. In such instances, the concentration of the suspect chemical in body fluids or tissues is very much greater than the concentration that would occur from trace environmental exposure.

More commonly, a person is concerned about the presence of environmental chemicals in his body. He wants to know where he can obtain an analysis for the presence of some synthetic chemical in his body. Often, the people most concerned are young mothers who want an analysis for some pesticide or other persistent chemical (e.g., PCBs or dioxins) in their breast milk. Anyone concerned about his or her body burden of an environmental chemical should ask, "Have I been exposed knowingly to the chemical?" Nursing mothers usually answer that they have not, but that they are concerned about nursing their babies after reading news stories telling of the contamination of mothers' milk.

The next question they should ask themselves is, "What am I going to do with the information, once I have it?" The usual answer to this question is that they do not know. They are often not aware that, in the absence of any unusual exposure to the chemical, a pretty good guess can be made as to what the analytic results would be, even without a laboratory analysis. It is important that young mothers know there are no known adverse effects in nursing babies from mothers' milk containing trace quantities of environmental chemicals. In addition, it is generally accepted that the immunologic and psychologic benefits of nursing far outweigh any unknown, subtle effect hypothesized for such chemicals.

An interesting point that may help give a perspective to today's young mothers is that if they were breast-fed babies, the chances are very good that the milk they received from their mothers had higher concentrations of such chemicals as DDT, PCBs, and dioxins than their own milk does now. Those chemicals are so much more rigorously controlled today than they were several decades ago that human exposures are now much lower.

Every one of us has trace quantities of chlorinated hydrocarbon chemicals stored within us—DDT, DDE, PCBs, dioxin, and so on. There is no known clinical significance that can be attached to trace quantities of these chemicals, or even to higher than average quantities of storage. Thus, there is no practical value in spending money for laboratory analyses to determine one's own body concentrations of these chemicals.

13

HUMAN EXPERIENCE

It is unfortunate that so much of the knowledge about the chronic effects of chemicals has come to us after the fact from illnesses of the people who worked with them. These people served as guinea pigs in the laboratory of human experience. Today, we would hope that society is more enlightened and that workers would not be permitted to be exposed to chemicals before the potential consequences of such exposure were known. The hope is fulfilled to the degree that now there are improved methods for studying the chronic effects of chemicals and that the public and government are aware that more must be known about these effects. As a result, laws have been enacted that require the conduct of chronic toxicity tests before large populations of people are knowingly exposed to potentially harmful chemicals.

However, we would be deceiving ourselves if we believed that scientific expertise, awareness of the problem, or laws requiring chronic toxicity testing can be as protective of working people as we would want them to be. This is not because of any lack of desire or motivation to protect workers, but rather because of the nature of toxicological science itself. No matter how much effort is put into the study of the chronic adverse effects of chemicals, and no matter how many studies yield negative results, one can never be sure that there is not some subtle effect that is yet to be discovered.

The importance of human data in evaluating the potential for adverse effects from exposure to chemicals, both acute and chronic, in the human population cannot be stressed too much. Whenever human data are available, they must take precedence over animal data in evaluating potential for human harm. After all, what animal model approximates human physiology and biochemistry more closely than the human itself? Unfortunately, data from human experience are largely ignored or rejected by people who are not experts in toxicology, particularly when the data indicate that humans are less sensitive than laboratory animals or when the matter becomes a political issue rather than a scientific one.

The most valuable human data come from tragic accidents or from mass exposures of people, either deliberately or inadvertently. There are so many of these episodes that only a few examples will be considered in this chapter.

DIOXINS—SEVESO, ITALY

The term *dioxin* has become a prominent entry in our lexicon of environmental pollutants. This is because dioxins, as contaminants in certain major industrial chemical products, are among the most toxic chemicals that have ever been synthesized, albeit inadvertently, by man. They were responsible for outbreaks of chick edema disease in the late 1950s that decimated large numbers of broiler flocks fed contaminated feed. They were responsible for the deaths during the early 1970s of many horses in a Times Beach, Missouri, horse farm where dioxin-contaminated oil was used to settle dust in arenas. They were the contaminants in the infamous herbicide Agent Orange blamed for numerous medical problems suffered by Vietnam veterans. An excellent review of dioxin releases into the environment and the copious literature on their health effects can be found in *Dioxin, Agent Orange, The Facts* by Michael Gough (1986. New York: Plenum Press).

Dioxins or chlorodibenzodioxins, as they are more properly called, are a class of compounds formed as by-product contaminants in a number of chemical reactions, including combustion. They are formed in trace quantities during the manufacture of some chlorinated aromatic organic compounds, such as 2,4,5-T (a component of the herbicide Agent Orange), trichlorophenol, or pentachlorophenol. Chlorodibenzodioxins are chlorine derivatives of the basic dibenzodioxin (DD) structure, which contains 12 carbon and 2 oxygen atoms.

The 12 carbons are arranged in two 6-carbon rings that are connected to each other by 2 oxygen bridges that join 2 adjacent carbons on one ring to 2 adjacent carbons on the other ring (see Figure 13–1). The DD structure can accept from 1 to 8 chlorine atoms—one chlorine for each of the carbons not tied up with oxygen. There are dozens of possible combinations of chlorine with DD. For example, there are 2 possible monochloro DDs, 10 possible dichloro DDs, 14 possible trichloro DDs, and so forth. However, there is only 1 octachloro DD because there is only one way to attach 8 chlorines to the 8 carbons in the DD structure.

Current environmental concerns about DDs center about their generation by a variety of human activities. The theory that chlorinated DDs and dibenzofurans (DFs) could be produced from chlorinated aromatic hydro-

Dibenzodioxin

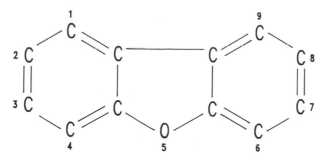

Dibenzofuran

Figure 13-1. Dibenzodioxin and dibenzofuran structures.

carbons by the action of heat or ultraviolet light was suggested 20 years ago by Donald G. Crosby, Department of Environmental Toxicology, University of California, Davis. Subsequently, the discovery that chlorinated DDs and DFs are produced in trace amounts during the combustion of solid-waste materials demonstrated that Dr. Crosby's hypothesis was correct.

The importance of these findings to the management of land and air quality is very great. The burning of organic materials produces trace quantities of dioxins in the environment, with the result that ambient air in populated areas contains traces of these chemicals. This background level of dioxin contamination, combined with the fact that rapidly dwindling sanitary landfill reserves mandates the development of alternate methods of solid waste disposal, has created a dilemma for local governments.

Recycling of dry materials, such as metal, plastic, glass, and paper, has become a serious endeavor is some communities. However, even if every household participated, recycling would eliminate only a small fraction of the garbage produced. One of the most cost-effective and efficient methods of waste disposal is conversion of waste to energy in power plants. In fact, such conversion plants are significant sources of revenue for the communities that have built them. However, public awareness that the process has the potential for producing chloro dioxins, even though it adds negligible quantities to background levels, has led to rejection of the process by some communities. Public fears of chloro dioxins far outweigh public concerns for the looming garbage crisis.

Toxicity studies of chloro DDs indicate that the intensity of their adverse effects increases from the monochloro derivatives up to the tetrachloro and then decreases from tetrachloro up to the octachloro compound. In the tetrachloro group, there is one that appears to occur more commonly than the others, namely 2,3,7,8-tetrachlorodibenzodioxin or TCDD for short. TCDD appears to be the most toxic of the chloro DDs.

In studies of acute toxicity of TCDD, the guinea pig is the most sensitive animal that has been discovered thus far. The oral LD_{50} for the guinea pig is between 0.6 and 4 $\mu g/kg$. The chicken appears to be the next most sensitive, with an oral LD_{50} between 25 and 50 $\mu g/kg$. All other animals—rats, mice, dogs, and so on—have oral LD_{50}'s between 100 and 200 $\mu g/kg$.

Chronic toxicity studies in monkeys show that 50 ppb TCDD in the diet causes death after 2 months, 5 ppb TCDD in about 6 months, and 0.5 ppb in about 11 months. TCDD is a potent teratogen in rats and mice, but it does not appear to be a teratogen in monkeys. It is too toxic in guinea pigs for successful conduct of teratogenicity studies in that species. The toxicity of TCDD shows wide variation among species not only in potency but also in the organ system involved. In humans, the only documented chronic toxic effect of TCDD is chloracne, a skin disease resembling the acne common to adolescence but much more persistent. There may be other less common effects in humans, such as liver damage or increased risk of certain cancers. However, there are not sufficient data to determine whether these cases are associated with TCDD or with the chemicals in which TCDD is a contaminant. Investigations of an association between TCDD exposure and adverse effects on the human reproductive process have been inconclusive.

The carcinogenicity of TCDD is difficult to assess. In animal studies, it appears to increase the incidence of some tumors and decrease the incidence of others. The fact that it influences the incidence of a variety of cancers supports the thesis that it is not a carcinogen but rather a cocarcinogen or promoter.

How might the data on the toxicity of TCDD obtained from animal experiments translate to man? If humans are as sensitive as the guinea pig, the acute lethal dose by ingestion for a 70-kg human would be 42 μg (70 kg $\times$ 0.6 $\mu g/kg$). If humans have a sensitivity like the majority of all other animals, the acute lethal dose would be between 7,000 and 14,000 μg.

Where does the human fit on the scale of sensitivity to TCDD? The tragedy of Seveso has helped provide us with some clues.

On July 10, 1976, a sudden and massive exposure of a whole town and all of its occupants, both human and animal, to TCDD occurred in Seveso, Italy. An accident in a plant that manufactured trichlorophenol, a chemical used in the production of the antiseptic, hexachlorophene, released reaction materials that contained 2 to 3 kg TCDD (some estimates run as high as 6 to 7 kg). The contamination covered an area of about 700 acres, with the heaviest concentration occurring in a 250-acre area. The unsuspecting population of tens of thousands in the surrounding community knew only that an explosion had occurred at the plant.

Within 6 days, 11 children were hospitalized with severe skin eruptions, which were eventually diagnosed as chloracne, a clinical symptom of exposure to TCDD. At about the same time, small animals—rabbits, chickens, wild birds—began dying. Then more children developed chloracne, and larger animals—dogs, sheep, cows, horses—began dying. In all, there were about 200 cases of chloracne, almost exclusively in children, and over 2,000 animal deaths. Finally, evacuation of the population was begun more than 2 weeks after the explosion, when soil and grass samples showed that very dangerous levels of TCDD were present in soils closest to the explosion. Some samples were found to be as high as 5,000 micrograms per square meter ($\mu g/m^2$).

The number of people involved in the zones around the plant that were judged to have high, moderate, and minimal exposures were approximately 750, 4,700, and 32,000, respectively. All of the women in the high- and moderate-exposure zones who were in their first 3 months of pregnancy were offered therapeutic abortions because of the knowledge that TCDD was a potent teratogen in animals. Of the approximately 150 women who were in their first trimester at the time of the accident, about 30 accepted the offer despite religious proscriptions against abortion. Among the 120 women who did not choose abortion, there were about 20 spontaneous abortions, a number not greater than normal.

When news of the accident became public, toxicologists around the world waited for the sad news of early 1977 when the first-trimester babies were due. Fortunately, there was no sad news. Of the just over 100 women who came to term, there were only 2 who bore children with anomalies, well within the normally expected number. One child had an intestinal obstruction and the other a genital malformation. Both malformations were corrected by surgery.

There is no information on the reasons for the spontaneous abortions; the numbers were overall within normal limits, but 1 or 2 percent higher in the high-exposure zone, a difference that was not statistically significant. It might have been expected that spontaneous abortions would have occurred in greater numbers than normal because of the great emotional stress of the situation. Examination of the abortus from the women choosing therapeutic abortion and of some that spontaneously aborted, although difficult to assess because of the trauma inflicted by the procedure, showed only one case of possible abnormality. That was a case suggestive of Down's syndrome, a defect that occurs at the time of conception. In this case, since conception was prior to the Seveso accident, it could not have been due to the accident.

The people of Seveso were away from their homes for a few months to several years while their government and the industry responsible for the accident tried to decide how to decontaminate their living areas. Homes in the high-contamination area remained contaminated for many years. TCDD penetrated the soil to a depth of almost a foot in the high-exposure zone. Chemical analyses of the soil of Seveso yielded values as high as 20,000 mg TCDD/acre. The lowest level of TCDD found in the 250 acres that were most highly contaminated was about 400 mg/acre. In addition, milk samples taken between 3 and 7 weeks after the accident from cows in the high-contamination zone contained from 1 to 7 ppb TCDD.

The people who moved back into their homes in Seveso are still being exposed to traces of TCDD. Since 1976, and for the rest of their lives, they will enact their involuntary roles as human guinea pigs. Their vital statistics, their chromosomes, their blood chemistry, their immunologic status, their cancer rates, and their general medical profiles have been and will continue to be of great interest to scientists worldwide. The British medical journal *Lancet* reported in the fall of 1982 that the town and surrounding area had not suffered dioxin poisoning, except for the chloracne cases in children. To date, there have been no observed chronic adverse effects from the tragedy that befell Seveso (Reggiani, G. M., The Seveso accident. In *Halogenated Biphenyls, Terphenyls, Naphthalenes, Dibenzodioxins and Related Products,* 2nd ed., R. D. Kimbrough and A. A. Jensen, eds., pp. 445–468. New York: Elsevier, 1989).

The final page will not be written until the people of Seveso and their children have lived out their lives. It is an important finding, however, that extremely high exposures to TCDD, for a period of more than 2 weeks' duration, to thousands of people of all ages and conditions, particularly pregnant women in the critical first trimester, had essentially no immediate adverse effect. No adverse chronic effects have been observed as of the latest report in 1989. The Seveso episode poses the very important question of why a chemical that is so extremely toxic to all animals, including the monkey, did not cause more immediate damage to a human population. It also points out that TCDD may be another chemical for which the monkey would not be an appropriate model for man.

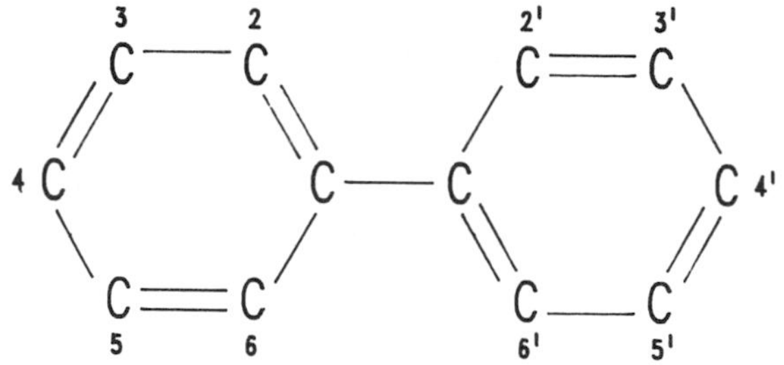

Figure 13-2. Biphenyl structure.

The human experience in Seveso tells us that the human being appears to be less susceptible to the adverse effects of TCDD than laboratory and domestic animals. It does not tell us that we should be any less cautious in our regulation of the compound—it is extremely toxic to many other species for which we must also be concerned.

PCBs AND DIBENZOFURANS— YUSHO DISEASE

Polychlorinated biphenyls (PCBs) are chlorinated aromatic hydrocarbon chemicals that have been in commercial use for over 50 years. Because of their physical and chemical properties they have found wide application as dielectric fluids in capacitors and transformers, heat transfer fluids, plasticizers, and general industrial fluids for engines and pumps. The PCB structure is based on biphenyl, a 12-carbon compound composed of two 6-member rings attached to each other by a carbon-to-carbon bond (see Figure 13-2). PCBs can accept from 1 to 10 chlorine atoms in their structures, 1 chlorine for each carbon designated by a number in Figure 13-2. There are over 200 possible combinations of biphenyl with chlorine. Commercial PCBs are not manufactured as pure compounds but rather as mixtures of chlorinated biphenyls. Their properties are dependent on the fraction of chlorine contained in the formulation. PCB formulations are identified by their chlorine content, which usually runs from between 20 and 70 percent. They are resistant to degradation and persist for long periods of time in the environment.

There is a wealth of data in the scientific literature on the toxic effects of PCBs. Acutely, PCBs are of a sufficiently low order of toxicity by all three routes of exposure to be classed as legally nontoxic. No toxicity studies have been performed on individual, purified isomers, but studies with mixtures of varying percent chlorine indicate that their toxicity increases with increasing degree of chlorination. PCBs also appear, from animal studies, to be of a relatively low order of toxicity chronically. There is evidence in the scientific literature that PCBs, like the majority of the chlorinated hydrocarbon compounds, produce liver tumors and occasionally liver cancers in rodent species. The significance of these findings for humans is questioned because the carcinogenic effect seems to be confined to rodent species.

There is evidence that at least part of the chronic toxicity of PCBs is due to impurities that occur in trace amounts in PCB formulations. These impurities, known as dibenzofurans (DFs), are relatives of the DDs, discussed above. DFs are composed of two 6-member carbon rings like DDs. However, unlike DDs, DF rings are joined together by one oxygen bridge and one carbon-to-carbon bond rather than two oxygen bridges. DFs contain 12 carbons and 1 oxygen (see Figure 13-1). Like DDs, DFs can accept up to 8 chlorine atoms, but they can form many dozens more possible combinations with chlorine than dioxin can because of the differences between the two in the way their 6-member rings are connected. Chlorinated DFs have not been the subject of as many studies as the chloro DDs. The data that are available indicate that chloro DFs are similar to chloro DDs in their mechanism of toxic action, but are from 10 to 1,000 times less toxic. For example, the guinea pig appears to be the animal most sensitive to TCDF (the chloro DF analogous to TCDD), as it is to TCDD, with an LD_{50} of 5 to 10 $\mu g/kg$. Other rodents have LD_{50}'s greater than 6,000 $\mu g/kg$. Despite the fact that chloro DFs are less toxic than chloro DDs, they may still be counted among the most highly toxic of synthetic compounds.

There have been a number of unfortunate accidents involving PCB contamination of foods. These episodes, in which humans have served as the involuntary guinea pigs, have provided toxicologists with the clinical symptomatology of subacute and chronic poisoning by PCBs in humans. One of the most extensively investigated and documented episodes of mass intoxication occurred in Japan in 1968. Several hundred people in one area of Japan became ill with an unknown disease whose symptoms included acnelike eruptions, swelling of the upper eyelids, hyperpigmentation of the mucous membranes, skin, and nails, and discharge from the eyes. The symptoms led to a tentative diagnosis of chloracne, and eventually the etiologic agent was found to be one particular brand of rice oil that was contaminated with PCBs. The disease became known as Yusho, which means "rice oil disease."

During the investigation into the cause of the illness, many more hundreds of people became ill with Yusho. The highest concentration of PCBs found in the rice oil was about 3,000 ppm. The chloro DF content of the PCB contaminant in the rice oil was calculated to be about 0.5 percent, which is equivalent to 5,000 ppm. Thus, rice oil containing 3,000 ppm PCB would contain chloro DF in an amount equal to 0.5 percent of 3,000 ppm, or about 15 ppm. This degree of chloro DF contamination is very much higher than normally found in commercial PCBs. Chloro DFs are usually present in PCBs in concentrations of less than 2 ppm, with the TCDF component being less than 0.05 ppm.

In the Yusho episode, the maximum quantity of contaminated oil consumed per person over a 3-month period was 4 to 5 liters. An investigation of the relationship between Yusho and the quantity of PCBs ingested led to the estimate that total doses of PCBs greater than 0.5 g, ingested over a several-month period, produced moderate to severe symptoms of Yusho disease. The maximum total dose of PCBs was calculated to be between 3 and 4 g.

More than 50 percent of the pregnant women who became ill with Yusho gave birth to infants with symptoms of the disease, indicating that PCBs (or the chloro DF contaminant) may be fetotoxic by ingestion. The possibility that some cases of infant illness were not the result of a direct toxic action on the fetus but rather of nonspecific illness secondary to poisoning in the mother cannot be ruled out. Yusho caused no deaths during the disease outbreak, with the possible exception of a few cases of stillbirths. No deaths have been attributed to the episode in the years since its occurrence. The people involved in the Yusho episode, like the people of Seveso, will be the subjects of medical surveillance for the rest of their lives. However, unlike the Seveso incident, the Yusho episode apparently has caused some cases of chronic illness (Kuratsune, M., Yusho, with reference to Yu-Cheng. In *Halogenated Biphenyls, Terphenyls, Naphthalenes, Dibenzodioxins and Related Products,* 2nd ed., R. D. Kimbrough and A. A. Allen, eds., pp. 381–400. New York: Elsevier, 1989).

The experience with Yusho cannot be translated directly to occupational exposures, because the former occurred with ingestion of PCBs and the exposure of working people is usually by inhalation or skin contact. The occurrence of chloracne in occupations using PCBs led to the establishment in 1942, about 13 years after the commercial introduction of the chemical, of a recommended maximum allowable concentration (MAC) for PCB in the workplace of 1 milligram per cubic meter of air (mg/m^3). About 15 years later, the recommended MAC for more highly chlorinated PCBs (54 percent chlorine) was lowered to 0.5 mg/m^3. The 1 mg/m^3 MAC was retained for the lesser chlorinated (42 percent) formulations.

Numerous epidemiologic surveys of people exposed for many years to PCBs in occupational settings have revealed essentially no adverse effects attributable to PCB exposure, other than occasional cases of chloracne and possibly diminished liver function. In 1977, the National Institute for Occupational Safety and Health (NIOSH) recommended that the permissible exposure level for PCBs in the workplace be reduced to one-thousandth of the current standard, from 1 mg/m^3 to 1 μg/m^3. The recommendation was based on an occasional finding of slightly elevated levels of certain liver enzymes in the blood of a few people exposed to PCBs, combined with the data on liver tumors produced in rodents by PCBs.

In its 1989 publication of recommended threshold limit values (TLVs, formerly referred to as MACs), the American Conference of Governmental Industrial Hygienists (ACGIH) still lists TLVs of 1 mg/m^3 and 0.5 mg/m^3 for PCBs. It has not added PCBs to its list of suspected human carcinogens, but it does note that the 54 percent chlorine PCBs have been identified by other sources as suspected human carcinogens.

In 1979, EPA prohibited the manufacture of PCBs in the United States and provided for severe restrictions and an orderly phaseout of its uses over a 5-year period. The ruling was deemed necessary because of its suspected carcinogenicity and its persistence in the environment. The full text of this important ruling appeared in the May 31, 1979, issue of the *Federal Register* (**44**:31,514–31,568). The cost–benefit ratio of the PCB ruling, an important aspect of such regulation usually ignored by the public, was made by the American Council on Science and Health ("PCBs: Is the Cure Worth the Cost?" revised May 1986).

Despite the ruling by EPA, PCBs will be with us for many years to come. The many decades of use of PCBs in transformers, capacitors, industrial machines and pumps, and so forth, has produced a tremendous number of machines and pieces of equipment containing PCBs that are still in use, and will be for many years to come. When replaced, they will be replaced with equipment that does not contain PCBs; in the meantime, the old equipment is subject to accident. Because they have a very long half-life in the environment, PCBs have become distributed in ppb or ppt quantities throughout the world.

It seems as though every day the news media contain reports of transformer explosions that spill "poisonous" PCBs over unsuspecting neighborhoods. Accidents involving PCBs must have occurred with the same regularity before PCBs were strictly regulated. However, since it was not known that they contained PCBs, such episodes were not newsworthy. PCB accidents certainly should not be treated lightly, and the people who clean up such spills should follow work practices that minimize their exposure. But public panic, engendered by scare reports issued by public officials who obviously have only the most superficial knowledge of the toxicology of PCBs and chloro DFs, is totally unnecessary. People who have been accidentally exposed to oils containing PCBs can remove the oils from themselves and their clothing with a good soapy washing. Furniture, automobiles, and other items can be washed to remove visible signs of contamination. After the episode is over, exposed individuals should *not* permit the contamination episode to become a source of worry and fear that they will develop cancer in 10 or 20 years.

There is absolutely no evidence that PCBs contaminated with trace quantities of DFs cause cancer in casually exposed humans. The best of this evidence is from epidemiologic studies of people whose jobs involved daily contact with PCBs. The absence of increased cancer rates in these groups makes it very difficult to believe that infrequent accidental exposures carry any cancer risk for the general public.

THE INSECTICIDE DDT

Dichloro diphenyl trichloroethane (DDT) was one of the first of a host of synthetic organic chemicals developed to fight insects. DDT was originally synthesized in 1874, but it was not until 1939 that its insecticidal properties were discovered in the Swiss laboratories of J. R. Geigy, by Paul Müller.

The first large-scale use of DDT occurred in January 1944, after several years of worldwide investigation of its effectiveness against insects and its toxicity to humans and animals. In December 1943, a typhus outbreak among the war refugees in Naples threatened to decimate the entire population of that Italian city. Within a month after the outbreak, the Allied forces began a DDT dusting program to combat the body louse, the vector of typhus. During January 1944, 1.3 million people were powdered with DDT at the rate of 10 pounds per 150 persons. By the time the dusting program was completed the disease was well under control. It was the first time in history that typhus had been controlled during winter months.

The great effectiveness of DDT in controlling all vector insects led to a decision by the Allied forces that was announced by Winston Churchill in a radio broadcast in September 1944: "The excellent DDT powder, which has been fully experimented with and found to yield astonishing results, will henceforth be used on great scale by the British forces in Burma and by the American and Australian forces in the Pacific and India in all theatres."

Thus began the worldwide distribution of DDT. Soldiers and civilians used it as a body and clothing powder to kill lice and ticks. Handfuls of DDT were tossed into rain barrels, cisterns, ponds, and lakes, all of which were used for drinking and bathing, to kill malaria mosquito larvae. DDT saved millions of lives from insect-borne diseases. It still continues to do so in third-world countries.

When the production of DDT finally exceeded the wartime demands for vector control, its use as a weapon against food crop pests began. The American Association of Economic Entomology heralded the extensive agricultural use of DDT that was to occur in the postwar years with the statement in September 1944 that ". . . never before in the history of entomology has a chemical been discovered that offers such promise to mankind for relief from his insect problem as DDT."

In 1948, Dr. Müller received the Nobel Prize in Medicine and Physiology for his discovery of DDT. In 1962, DDT was brought to public attention as the maleficent star of Rachael Carson's best-selling book *Silent Spring* (Boston: Houghton Mifflin). From that year, until it was finally banned by EPA in 1972, DDT was decried as the scourge of our planet. What trick of fate transformed DDT from Winston Churchill's "excellent powder" into Rachel Carson's "elixir of death"?

The answer lies in the age-old adage that hindsight is better than foresight. It was known that DDT was highly resistant to degradation and that it was stored in body fat of organisms exposed to it, but the full significance of these properties for its spread throughout the world was beyond the scientific sophistication of the 1940s. In addition, the stimulus that DDTs success gave to the field of synthetic organic chemistry spurred significant improvements in analytical chemical methods. These refinements enabled chemists to detect quantities of DDT (or PCBs—see above) in ppm quantities, thereby revealing to Ms. Carson and other scientists the extent of DDT spread in the environment.

The environmental movement received tremendous impetus, if not actual birth, from Ms. Carson's book. Laboratory analyses demonstrated that DDT was virtually omnipresent throughout the world. The decline in populations of wildlife species, such as the brown pelican and perigrine falcon, were attributed to environmental contamination by DDT. The campaign to ban DDT was initiated. The publicity accompanying the campaign gave rise to widespread fears that people, too, were being harmed by DDT. The campaign was successful. The use of DDT was banned in the United States within 10 years. It became a fact that DDT was responsible for wildlife declines, and attention turned to other persistent pesticides.

Shortly after the ban on DDT use, ecologists and environmentalists stopped pointing to DDT as a hazard to the health of wild creatures. By 1977, numerous stories began appearing in the public press about the return of brown pelicans and perigrine falcons. In 1984, NRDC reported that DDT was the most commonly found pesticide in California produce. In 1989, the Sierra Club announced that the brown pelican, large colonies of which have returned to the California coast, was no longer on the endangered species list. Today, residues of DDT are still found in air, fresh and sea water, fish and other marine organisms, and birds taken from all around the world. The continued presence of DDT in the environment is attributed primarily to its continued use by third-world and Eastern-bloc countries. If DDT was the cause of decline of certain species, why have those species returned in the face of continued environmental contamination with DDT? The answer to this question is essential not to vindicate DDT but to gain a better understanding of the complex interplay between environmental pollution and environmental health.

Predictions that environmental contamination by DDT would cause an increase in cancer incidence have not been fulfilled. In a paper entitled "Chemical Carcinogens in the Environment and in the Human Diet: Can a Threshold Be Established?" Claus and co-workers examined the practical application of one risk-estimate formula to DDT exposure:

> If one . . . examines the exposures to DDT which would be "unsafe," accepting the 10^{-6} safety factor for man suggested by Schneiderman (1970) and applying his preferred curve, a serious problem emerges. According to his method, the exposure which should cause tumours in 1 in 100 individuals (TD_1) is a total dose of 30 ng/man/day. In view of the fact that the whole human population of the earth has been ingesting at least 1000 times this quantity of pesticide daily for the past 25 years, one would expect that were DDT indeed carcinogenic for man, and were these safety assumptions based in reality, there ought to have been a massive increase in primary liver cancer among humans in the age group at highest risk, that is, in those who are now between 50 and 70 years old. In effect, the average daily intake of DDT by man over these 25 years would correspond approximately to Schneiderman's TD_{50} and thus, in the population at risk, exposed for at least a quarter of their lives, every eighth person should have developed hepatocarcinoma. (*Food and Cosmetics Toxicology* **12**:737, 1974).

This example is even more striking when one considers that liver cancer is sufficiently uncommon and that it is often grouped in the catch-all category of "All Other Cancers" in compilations of cancer morbidity and mortality statistics. It is estimated that liver cancer represents only 4 percent of all cancers in the United States. There is no evidence that DDT is a human carcinogen.

INDOOR AIR POLLUTION

Indoor air pollution has become a common problem for modern society. The adverse health effects attributed to indoor air pollution are referred to as tight building syndrome and sick building syndrome. Indoor air pollution is included in this section, because it represents another complex environmental health problem that affects a large number of people. Beginning in the early 1970s, increasing numbers of complaints and reports of illness from office workers called attention to this new health problem associated with indoor air quality. It differs from typical occupational health problems in that it is most often not caused by one or two airborne contaminants but usually by a large mixture of trace quantities of pollutants, none of which alone appears capable of causing illness.

Illnesses associated with office buildings were recognized many years before indoor air pollution was identified as the cause. The Bateson Building, a State of California office building in Sacramento that opened its doors to its first occupants in 1981, is an early example in which the relationship between indoor air pollution and illness was readily apparent. This new building was the realization of a much-publicized effort to create a State building that would serve as a model for the ultimate in energy conservation. Within a year, the monument to energy efficiency was the target of a $500,000 class action suit in behalf of the 1,200 employees in the building. Their suit was based on the claim that working in the building made people ill. A survey by an employee organization showed that 80 percent of the employees on one floor of the building had one or more symptoms that they attributed to the building environment. Their symptoms included various ailments of the upper and lower respiratory tracts, nausea, itching or burning eyes, sinus problems, skin irritation, dizziness, and fainting spells. An engineering survey concluded that the ventilation system was providing inadequate fresh air circulation.

The problems found in buildings such as the Bateson Building are most often caused by poor ventilation that leads to an accumulation of a wide range of air pollutants in the building. Most frequently, investigations show that indoor air pollution is composed of airborne gases, vapors, particles, odors, and exhaled air that have been released inside the building by structural materials, clothing, people, office products, office furnishings, and smoking. Less frequently noted contaminants are chemicals and solvents from office reproduction equipment, products of combustion from stoves and furnaces, and growths of fungi and other microorganisms in wet areas of the building or its ventilation system.

Occasionally polluted air enters the fresh air intakes of the ventilation system from outside the building. These outside pollutants are usually automobile exhaust, cooling tower mists, products of combustion from nearby smokestacks, or air pollutants from nearby industry. The majority of problems, however, are caused by the buildup of airborne contaminants as the result of energy-saving building designs that restrict the intake of fresh air to conserve energy. In some cases, only parts of the building are poorly ventilated. In other cases, the ventilation system is adequate, but poorly maintained or operated.

The problems caused by microbial contamination deserve further mention because of the serious illnesses and deaths that sometimes occur. One example, the outbreak of Legionnaires' disease in a Philadelphia building in 1976, resulted in 182 cases and 29 deaths due to acute respiratory infections. The cause was traced to airborne *Legionnella* bacteria. This is an example of a general class of an often serious but infrequent indoor air pollution problem. In these cases, bacteria, fungi, or other microorganisms contaminate and then multiply in cooling tower water, in stagnant wet areas inside ventilation systems, or in wet carpets or furnishings. With the right conditions these organisms will become airborne and be dispersed by the building ventilation system. The resulting effects depend on the organism involved.

Prevention depends on the elimination of potential sources of microbial contamination of building intake air, and control of microbial growth within the building by controlling stagnant water accumulation in ventilation systems or on carpets and furnishings. In addition to pathogen-borne diseases, a variety of disorders, such as hypersensitivity pneumonitis, humidifier fever, allergic rhinitis, and conjunctivitis, have been reported.

In 446 episodes of tight building syndrome investigated by the National Institute for Occupational Safety and Health (NIOSH), the primary causes have been classified as follows (*Indoor Air Quality.* Cincinnati: NIOSH, Sept. 1989):

- Inadequate ventilation, 52%
- Contamination from inside the building, 17%
- Contamination from outside the building, 11%
- Microbiological contamination, 5%
- Contamination from the building fabric, 3%
- Unknown, 12%

Anyone who has been affected by indoor air pollution or who wants to learn how to conduct an investigation of indoor air quality should obtain a copy of the NIOSH publication *Indoor Air Quality,* mentioned above.

What are the pollutants in indoor air? Studies have identified many of the contaminants as chemicals originating from the occupants, furniture, structural materials, cleaning and polishing materials, and office machinery. Many other chemicals in indoor air are not known and may never be identified. The composition of indoor air pollution is almost infinitely variable. The fact that inadequately ventilated rooms made people ill long before the advent of the petrochemical industry suggests that stoves and furnaces, pathogens (viruses, bacteria, molds), natural allergens (pollens, animal dander, etc.), tobacco smoke, and even the products of human metabolism exhaled from the lungs or excreted in their sweat were significant factors. The suggestion has even been made that the buildup of radon, a naturally occurring radioactive gas given off by soils and rocks and by building materials made from them, in unventilated rooms also contributes to illness. Of all of the chemicals from human sources, carbon monoxide has the greatest potential for causing illness, or even death, because it has the greatest potential for achieving dangerous air concentrations from inadequate ventilation of combustion sources.

The use of synthetic materials in construction and furniture and the use of organic chemicals in office supplies and equipment have added to the burden of indoor air pollution. Probably the one chemical that has caused people the most difficulty is formaldehyde. Formaldehyde is a simple organic chemical containing only one carbon atom. It is widely distributed in nature and is present in all of us as a product of the metabolism of one-carbon biochemicals. It is also used extensively in the plastics and polymer industry.

Formaldehyde is an extremely irritating gas that is intolerable in concentrations greater than a few ppm in air. Preserving solutions for biologic and pathologic materials are usually 3.7 percent formaldehyde. Solutions of formaldehyde are irritating to skin, eyes, and mucous membranes. Formaldehyde is a strong sensitizer, and the usual symptoms that people develop from exposure to formaldehyde vapors are those of an allergic nature. These symptoms include skin rashes, headache, puffy eyes, and respiratory problems. It has been estimated that perhaps 10 percent of the population is allergic to formaldehyde. The people at greatest risk of adverse effect from exposure to formaldehyde are those who work with concentrated solutions, such as chemical workers, undertakers, pathologists, and other scientists who work with preserved biological specimens. Their exposure is many orders of magnitude greater than that which occurs in indoor air pollution.

The carcinogenicity of formaldehyde has been given a great deal of attention by the news media; thus, any mention of the effects of exposure to formaldehyde would be incomplete without reference to its carcinogenicity:

> Formaldehyde gas is carcinogenic for rats and probably for mice, producing nasal tumors after inhalation. Limited experiments in Syrian hamsters have not demonstrated carcinogenicity. In rats, the carcinogenic response appears nonlinear, being disproportionately higher at higher concentrations. (Occupational exposure to formaldehyde: Final rule. *Federal Register* 52(233):46,205, Dec. 4, 1987).

Animal studies give no evidence that formaldehyde causes cancer in any site other than the nasal passages. In humans, some epidemiological studies of occupational groups show no association between exposure to formaldehyde and cancer incidence. In other studies a weak association is seen. Therefore, although formaldehyde remains a suspected human carcinogen, it is important for the public to recognize that the concentrations encountered in indoor air pollution are very much smaller than the occupational exposures that are of concern in the studies of cancer risk from exposure to formaldehyde. The allergenic properties of formaldehyde are of much greater significance to the general public than its potential carcinogenicity. A review of the extensive data on the health effects of formaldehyde can be found in OSHA's final rule on formaldehyde, cited above.

Many articles, both popular and scientific, have been written on the phenomenon of indoor air pollution in which it is treated as a new problem created by modern society. Probably even before the beginnings of ventilation engineering science, and well before the use of synthetic chemicals in structural materials and home furnishings, it was known that you could not close up people in airtight rooms without making them ill. The widespread publicity about indoor air pollution has created a growing public demand for more information about the causes of the problem.

In response to demands for stricter governmental controls, new bureaucracies have been formed to study and regulate indoor air pollution. The environmental science departments of colleges and universities have added indoor air pollution to their curricula. National and international organizations dedicated to the subject have come into being. Millions of dollars of public and private money are being invested in indoor air pollution research. A new science has been born! A new industry and a new occupation also have been born—indoor air pollution control and indoor air pollution inspectors.

Indoor air pollution is an excellent example of two principles that are exhibited so often during the implementation of advances in science and technology. The first is that solution of one problem often creates another, possibly more severe, problem. The second is that, throughout history, the figurative wheel keeps being reinvented. In accordance with the first principle, indoor air pollution is the problem created by the attempt to solve the problem of the high cost and shortage of energy. In order to reduce the expenditure of energy necessary to provide a comfortable indoor air environment, buildings are made more airtight to keep the warmed indoor air from escaping. At the same time, energy is saved by eliminating the need to heat or cool new fresh replacement air from the outdoors. Fuel is saved, and people are made ill.

In the second principle, the solution to the problem of how to keep people from being made ill in modern, fuel-efficient buildings may be symbolized by the proverbial wheel. There is a massive effort underway to solve the problem, when the solution is already at hand—the wheel has already been invented. It does not need reinventing. Ventilation engineering technology developed all of the formulas used to calculate the proper number of air changes required for healthful air quality many years ago. The solution to the problem of indoor air pollution is adequate air exchange. More research may be needed to devise methods for conserving energy while providing for adequate air exchange, but no more research is needed to prevent adverse effects from indoor air pollution.

The composition of indoor air pollution will probably continue to be researched for many years to come because of its importance to public health. A great deal of information may be added to the fund of scientific knowledge. Will any practical solution, other than the one that is already known, come from the tremendous amount of time, effort, and money that is currently being spent on the problem? At some time in the distant future, when and if all of the facts are finally known, the answer to the problem will probably be the one that is already at hand. That answer, which comes from the wisdom of ventilation engineers, is to provide adequate numbers of air exchanges in all buildings, public and private.

14

EPIDEMIOLOGY

Epidemiology is the study of the occurrence and movement of diseases in groups of people and the investigation of the relationships of these diseases to causative factors. The purpose of epidemiology is to describe the symptoms of a particular disease and to discover the chain of association between the disease and its etiological (causative) agent. Epidemiology may be termed the science of search methods. Along with logical thinking and systematic documentation, epidemiology makes use of a number of scientific specialties, such as clinical medicine, pathology, biochemistry, and bacteriology, to collect and evaluate data on health effects. Biostatistical methods are used to look for and evaluate associations between effects and possible causes.

The science of epidemiology arose out of interest in learning the cause of the epidemics of diseases, such as bubonic plague, typhus, and cholera, that swept through Europe and Asia prior to the end of the nineteenth century, leaving huge death tolls in their wake. Early epidemiologists, by systematically observing and recording exactly who contracted a particular disease and who did not, where, when, and under what conditions, were able to obtain sufficient information about cause and effect to prevent some epidemics despite the fact that the specific etiologic agent was not even suspected, much less identified.

ORIGINS OF MODERN EPIDEMIOLOGY

John Snow, an English physician, is one of the pioneers of modern epidemiology. Snow studied outbreaks of cholera in London during the middle of the nineteenth century. At that time, cholera was a common disease that regularly devastated large populations of people throughout Europe and Asia. The disease seemed to spread from person to person, but how or why was a mystery. Snow recognized that cholera was associated with poverty, overcrowding, refuse, and filth. He also suspected that the distribution of cholera cases in London was somehow associated with the source of drinking water. The frequency of cases seemed to increase with increasing sewage contamination of the water supply.

When an outbreak of cholera occurred in 1848 in a small section of London known as the Golden Square, Snow systematically identified and then plotted each case of cholera on a spot map of the area. The spot map showed that most of the cholera cases were centered around one water pump known as the Broad Street pump. Further investigation of cholera cases among the population living in Golden Square at the time also showed that there were two groups that had a very low incidence of the disease. One group was a workhouse population of over 500 inhabitants that used water from the workhouse well rather than the Broad Street pump. The other group was a population of 70 workers in a brewery. In checking the drinking water source used by brewery workers, Dr. Snow learned that the workers most likely drank no water at all from the surrounding community; workers were provided with free ale. In addition, the brewery had a deep well of its own. Dr. Snow went on to study the number of cases of cholera among the customers of two competing water companies that drew water from different areas of the Thames River. Again his results showed that water polluted with sewage was associated with cholera.

Despite these careful studies, Dr. Snow's findings did not indicate that cholera was transmitted by a pathogen in the water. In fact, the concept that microorganisms could transmit disease had not yet been formulated. However, he did show a strong association between water contaminated with sewage and the incidence of the disease cholera. This information alone was extremely important, because it gave direction to practical preventive programs and further studies aimed at finding the causative agent. In fact, based on Dr. Snow's investigations, the development of sanitary procedures to keep drinking water free of contamination by sewage virtually eliminated cholera. However, the final proof of the cause–effect relationship did not come until years later when the infectious organism was isolated, identified, and demonstrated to be the actual cause of the disease.

Epidemiology is a rigorous discipline that relies heavily on biostatistical methodology. A competent epidemiologist must not only be well-founded in medical, biological, and statistical sciences but must also be an imaginative and curious detective. The latter qualities are essential to uncover and properly weigh all of the many factors that might be associated with the problem under investigation.

EPIDEMIOLOGY OF NONINFECTIOUS DISEASES

Before proceeding, it is important to comment on the common impression that the biostatistical component of an epidemiologic study can reveal the cause of a disease. This false concept has led to a great deal of public confusion and dissatisfaction with epidemiologic investigations of cancer and birth defect clusters. For example, in a community where a cluster exists, community fatality and/or illness records are sifted for possible associations with environmental factors, such as water source, pesticide use, or socioeconomic status. These investigations may or may not indicate an association.

If there is no statistical association, there is probably no cause–effect relationship. A weak association may be suggestive, but it cannot be used immediately for preventive purposes. An association is most useful when it is very strong. For example, if a disease has almost no occurrence in a non-exposed group, and a high occurrence in an exposed group, the association between the disease and the exposure is very strong. However, cause–effect relationships can only be proven when all of the components that make up a valid and complete epidemiologic study support such a relationship. These components include accurate diagnosis, biostatistically significant differences in comparable population groups, identification of etiological agent, and evidence of exposure. The key point is that while biostatistical studies may contribute valuable information, they are only one step in the epidemiologic process. People must recognize that the biostatistical component of a study can only demonstrate associations.

Epidemiology had its origins a century ago in the study of infectious diseases where it was of great value. Today, lung cancer and heart disease are the important causes of disability and death. These are noninfectious diseases associated with life-style patterns, nutritional factors, age, and chemicals. Experience has been that epidemiologic investigations of these diseases are much more difficult than investigations of infectious diseases. The reasons are many. Early symptoms are often silent or vague, latency periods are usually measured in years rather than days, and the diseases in question tend to have some normal rate of occurrence throughout the general population. The result is that associations are not easily apparent.

Extensive use of biostatistics is often required to learn (1) whether the rate of disease in the group in question is higher than the normal background level and (2) whether the disease is associated with any common factors within the group. Without a significant association from the biostatistical studies, further steps in the epidemiologic investigative process are not usually taken. Unfortunately, weak or suggestive associations are often cited in various popular reading materials as proof of a cause–effect relationship.

Epidemiology, nevertheless, is a most valuable, and often essential, adjunct to investigations of the beneficial or adverse effects of chemicals in human populations. The populations of interest to toxicologists are those that may suffer adverse effects from exposure to specific chemicals. They may be groups of people who work at the same occupation and, thus, have the same exposure to an industrial chemical, or they may be groups of people who live in the same community and, thus, share the same exposure to some environmental contaminant in their air or water supply.

One approach that epidemiologists use is to compare two groups of people that are as alike as possible with the exception of their exposure to a specific chemical. Another approach is to compare two groups that are as alike as possible with the exception of their incidence of a specific disease. These methods use what is known as matched populations. The first method compares people with differences in exposure to the chemical in question and looks for differences in incidence of the disease. The second method compares people with differences in incidence of the disease and looks for differences in exposure to the chemical. The rationale for these approaches is that if the chemical under investigation does cause a specific disease, that disease will occur with greater frequency in the groups exposed to the chemical.

Epidemiologic studies may be retrospective or prospective. Retrospective studies look back on populations exposed in the past. Prospective studies look forward to populations that will be exposed in some future time. Retrospective studies suffer from the fact that critical data—that is, what dose of chemical did each person receive and for how long a period of time— are often not available or cannot be retrieved because the time is past. Such data must be estimated, a procedure fraught with uncertainty and error.

Prospective studies do not suffer from such uncertainties. Plans are made in advance to record levels and times of exposure, health status prior to exposure, and so forth. Thus, properly designed prospective studies usually yield valuable information on chronic effects of chemicals. In recent years, a number of the major companies in the chemical industry have instituted programs of prospective epidemiology among their employees for all new chemicals they manufacture and for some of the older ones that have come under suspicion as being a cause of health problems. The major deficiency of prospective epidemiologic investigations is that the answers being sought are not forthcoming immediately. In some cases, it may take many years to evaluate fully the significance for health of chronic exposure to a chemical.

As mentioned previously, it is important to recognize that the key word is *association*. Statistical analyses can only reveal whether or not two factors are related and, if so, how strongly. No matter how strong the association between two factors, the relationship is not necessarily a causal one.

For example, several decades ago, before it became fashionable for women to wear pants or slacks, an almost perfect association could be demonstrated between the wearing of skirts and the incidence of breast cancer. Another example of a strong correlation between unrelated occurrences is the decline in the stork population in Europe accompanied by a decline in birth rate. Despite the very strong associations, no one would claim that the wearing of skirts caused breast cancer or that storks brought babies.

These amusing examples do not in any way lessen the very great value of statistical analyses in the study of the relationship between disease and exposure to chemicals. However, they do serve as a warning to the public to be very wary of any study that claims to prove a cause–effect relationship based on statistics alone.

If a study does show a relationship between an environmental contaminant and a disease cluster, further work is required to demonstrate a cause–effect connection, no matter how strong the association. The model for determining cause–effect relationship for infectious diseases was first applied in 1876 by Robert Koch, a German physician. These criteria, known as *Koch's Postulates,* may be summarized as follows:

1. The organism responsible for the disease must be present in every case of the disease.
2. The organism must be isolated from the patients and grown in pure culture.
3. The organism grown in pure culture must be able to cause the disease in a healthy host.
4. The organism must be recovered again from the experimentally infected host.

Koch's postulates cannot be directly applied to environmental chemicals because of the differences between microorganisms and chemicals in how they cause diseases. However, the postulates are very useful in helping to illustrate the new and difficult problems faced by investigators who study the causes of noninfectious diseases.

Postulate 1: The organism responsible for the disease must be present in every case of the disease. When considering environmental chemicals, all people with the disease in question may not have been exposed to the suspected chemical. Many of the diseases caused by chemicals are the same as those that have a normal background incidence in the general population. Leukemia is a good example. It is known to be caused by ionizing radiation and by benzene, but it also has a measurable background incidence in the general population. Thus, the investigator searching for causes of leukemia in population groups must take into account the possible contribution of several environmental agents as well as a background level of the disease.

Postulate 2: The organism must be isolated from the patients and grown in pure culture. It may be difficult or impossible to obtain the chemical in pure form from the patient. Chemicals are often metabolized and excreted in different form. Adverse health effects may be the result of a combination of chemicals. Some of the chemicals may be unstable and difficult to isolate. The components of the mixture may vary over time, as is the case with polluted air or contaminated water.

Postulate 3: The organism grown in pure culture must be able to cause the disease in a healthy host. It is possible to translate this to a postulate that states that the suspected chemical or chemicals in pure form must be able to cause the symptoms in appropriate animal (or other) models. The problem with this postulate is that causation of disease by chemicals is dose-dependent. High doses often cause different symptoms and effects than low doses. Further, measuring the effects of low doses of chemicals in a host animal requires a long time and a great many animals. On the other hand, measuring the ability of an organism grown in pure culture to cause an infectious disease in a healthy host animal is a relatively straightforward process.

Postulate 4: The organism must be recovered again from the experimentally infected host. This could be translated to say that the mechanism of causation must be elucidated and some evidence of the suspected chemical (the chemical itself, a metabolic product, etc.) must be found in the affected subjects. Demonstration of the biochemical mechanism whereby a chemical causes a disease is probably the most important step in proving a cause-effect relationship.

Despite all the problems and complexities involved in proving a true cause-effect relationship, it must be stressed that none of the above steps are essential for instituting preventive measures if there is reason to suspect that a chemical is doing human or environmental damage. As illustrated by Dr. Snow, practical preventive measures can be derived from strong association between environmental factors and incidence of disease. This is particularly true for chemicals that affect small numbers of people or take many years to show an effect because scientific proof is often difficult or impossible to obtain. This problem will be explored further in the discussion on trans-science (Chapter 16).

STUDY DESIGN—PRECEPTS AND PITFALLS

Epidemiologists are guided by procedures based on sound principles that have been developed through the many decades since the time of Dr. Snow and his colleagues. However, there is no cookbook that sets forth the details of an epidemiologic study design. Every situation is unique. The value of the results obtained from an epidemiologic study will depend on the competence of the study design and the resources available for proper conduct of the study. There are numerous factors that must be considered in the design and conduct of a study. Examples of a few factors and the difficulties that they can present in the study of noninfectious agents are mentioned below.

Perhaps one of the greatest difficulties in designing an epidemiologic study is recognizing and accounting for all of the possible factors that might be associated with a disease under investigation. This is a particular problem in modern society with diseases of unknown etiology. Populations are so diverse, particularly in the United States with its many cultures and ethnic groups, that many patterns of exposure can exist within a narrow geographical area. The epidemiologist must consider not only the more usual common exposures, such as air and water, but also occupational exposures, dietary habits, unique drugs or medical treatments, hobbies and crafts, and recreational activities. If some critical factor related to the disease is unknown or unsuspected, an epidemiologic investigation is unlikely to reveal its association with the disease.

Outbreaks of neonatal jaundice in the Imperial Valley of California several decades ago provide a good example of how lack of complete information can interfere in the resolution of a problem. Neonatal jaundice is a disease that occurs among newborn infants as a result of a normal physiological process. During uterine life, the fetus has smaller amounts of oxygen available to it from mother's blood than it will have from its own lungs after birth. The fetus compensates by making extra red blood cells to carry oxygen. After birth, it does not need as many red cells, so the excess cells are destroyed. The hemoglobin in the destroyed cells is degraded to bilirubin, a pigment that gives the skin, mucous membranes, and whites of the eyes a yellow color. Destruction of old or excess red blood cells is a normal occurrence in humans, but adults have liver enzyme systems that rapidly destroy bilirubin and excrete it in the bile. These enzymes are either lacking or not present in sufficient quantities at birth. Perhaps as many as half of newborn infants develop mild visible signs of jaundice.

The Imperial Valley episode occurred in the early 1960s. Excess cases of serious neonatal jaundice occurred in babies born during the late summer months in a relatively new hospital surrounded by an agricultural area where a large amount of cotton was grown. Similar outbreaks had occurred each year during the same months for the several prior years. Because of their extensive use in the agricultural area surrounding the hospital, pesticides came under suspicion as the cause of the outbreaks. Hospital records showed that the number of cases of neonatal jaundice increased among babies born at about the same time that cotton defoliants were sprayed on the surrounding acres of cotton. Thus, a possible cause was that the defoliant was causing liver damage in the newborns which, in turn, was causing jaundice by preventing the breakdown of excess bilirubin.

Inspection of the hospital, which was new and modern, with few exterior windows, revealed no conditions within the hospital that prevailed only during the late summer months. Surveys of other hospitals in the same agricultural area showed no excess cases of neonatal jaundice, despite the facts that cotton defoliants and other agricultural chemicals were used to the same extent in the same months as in the vicinity of the affected hospital. Although the association with cotton defoliation was strong in the affected hospital, application of sound epidemiologic principles indicated that the relationship was not with agricultural chemicals.

Independently in England, an observant nurse noted that newborn babies in cribs near sunlit windows were less likely to suffer neonatal jaundice than infants in the interior of the nursery (Fincher, J., Notice: Sunlight may be necessary for your health, *Smithsonian,* pp. 71–76, June 1985). Subsequent clinical investigation of the nurse's observation revealed that the degradation of bilirubin in newborns is hastened by exposure to bright daylight. Since the late 1960s, the routine treatment for neonatal jaundice has been exposure of affected babies to bright artificial light.

In retrospect, it seems so obvious that the excess cases of neonatal jaundice and the spraying of cotton defoliants in the Imperial Valley many years ago were also associated with the hottest summer months, when people of all ages stay indoors as much as possible to avoid sunlight. The fact that the hospital had few windows compared to other hospitals in the area was thought unimportant at the time. However, the lack of windows combined with the propensity to keep newborns inside during the hot summer months reduced their exposure to daylight to the point where they could not degrade their bilirubin at a rate sufficient to avoid jaundice. The clinical demonstration of the causal relationship between bright light and bilirubin destruction supports a theory that the Imperial Valley cases were due to a lack of bright light rather than liver disease caused by exposure to cotton defoliants.

Another difficulty in designing epidemiologic studies of noninfectious agents is in grouping symptoms and counting numbers of cases. It is important that apples not be counted as oranges, unless there is a valid reason to do so. How to group cases is a major problem in studying cancer clusters. Cancer is not a single disease. It may be as many as a hundred different diseases with a hundred different causes. In most cancer clusters, there is usually not just one type of cancer represented. There may be cases of cancer of the brain, kidneys, bone, lymph system, and so forth. This poses a problem for biostatisticians; the fewer the number of cases of a single disease, the more data required to demonstrate an association with some environmental agent.

Is it valid to consider different cancers as the same disease in order to increase the number of cases in a cancer cluster? It is valid *only* if the environmental agent under investigation is capable of causing all different kinds of cancer, such as is the case with ionizing radiation. With few exceptions, carcinogenic chemicals are not random in their effects; they cause specific cancers. Therefore, it is seldom valid to group different cancers when looking for an association with a chemical agent. Unfortunately, this is a difficult concept for the public to understand. It is one that news stories usually ignore.

The collection of data is an especially important and sensitive aspect of a study design. Probably the least reliable method of obtaining information from people is by questionnaires that solicit information in the absence of an experienced interviewer. Such questionnaires ask about symptoms, history of illnesses, and history of exposures. Responses are difficult to evaluate because people differ in their ability to recall. They may not have the same understanding of the questions, and their perceptions of the severity of symptoms may be tempered by their ability to tolerate illness.

A valid epidemiologic study cannot be conducted from the comfort of an office. The people who design a study and collect and evaluate the data obtained should go into the field to see the situation firsthand. They must talk to the people involved. They must explain the study and what its problems and potentials are. As was the case with the English nurse and the newborn infants with neonatal jaundice, people involved on the scene often have knowledge or make observations that are critical to the outcome of the investigation.

Information about the normal frequency of a disease in a population is essential before any determination can be made that its incidence is increasing or decreasing. Such information comes from statistics on morbidity and mortality, which often may not be as reliable as desired. If there is no normal occurrence of a disease in a population, the epidemiology of cases that do occur is simplified. For example, cholera has no normal background incidence in the United States because of good sanitation practices. Thus, an outbreak of cholera in this country would be quickly noted and the cause would be relatively easy to find.

However, for noninfectious chronic diseases such as cardiovascular diseases and cancer there are background levels in all populations. The epidemiology of cancer and cardiovascular disease involves small differences in background incidence between populations or small changes within a population; hence the great importance of a knowledge of what the background is. In recent decades considerable data have been collected on age, sex, and geographic distributions of cancer and heart disease. These data provide the very valuable data bank required for epidemiologic studies of their association with environmental factors.

The importance of a knowledge of normal disease patterns to the interpretation of data obtained from epidemiologic studies can be seen in studies of the relationship between exposure to pesticides and the incidence of cancer. There is an intuitive conviction among people and even among some health officials that exposure to trace quantities of pesticides must be causing some disease. As a result, numerous studies have been conducted to compare cancer incidence between rural (presumed pesticide-exposed) and urban (presumed not pesticide-exposed) populations. A usual finding is a slightly greater incidence of certain leukemias and lymphomas among rural residents than urban residents, despite the fact that overall cancer rates are higher in urban populations. A knowledge of the literature on differences in morbidity and mortality between rural and urban populations is essential for an evaluation of these data.

Studies of vital statistics from years prior to 1960, and as early as 1943, in California, other parts of the United States, and in other countries, indicated that certain leukemias and lymphomas had a higher incidence in rural areas than in urban areas. Elfriede Faisal, a physician and medical epidemiologist with the California Department of Public Health, observed from these and her own studies that the differences were probably real and associated with exposure to the farm environment (*American Journal of Epidemiology,* **87**(2):267–274, 1968). The data reported in Dr. Faisal's paper were obtained in years prior to extensive use of synthetic pesticides in agriculture. In fact, many of the pesticides in current agricultural use were not commercially available prior to 1960. Studies designed to investigate adverse effects of exposure to any agent must consider data from preexposure studies for proper interpretation.

As with any science, epidemiology can be misused. Misuses usually involve efforts to support preconceived opinions concerning causal, or lack of causal, relationships. Even with the best of intentions, studies can be incomplete or faulty. It is very difficult for the average person to evaluate critically data obtained from epidemiologic investigations. Since prevention of disease is the ultimate goal of epidemiology, biased or incompetent studies are, at best, wasteful of resources, and, at worst, detrimental to the public welfare. They do not provide information that can help in disease prevention, and they may needlessly mislead or inflame the public.

UNREASONABLE EXPECTATIONS

It has become very popular in recent years for public agencies to employ epidemiologic techniques to investigate the relationship between the health status of a population and contaminants in air, food, or water. Such studies are a proper function of public agencies, and a great deal of excellent and valuable information can come from them if they are well-designed, carefully planned, and conducted by professional epidemiologists. In fact, much of our knowledge of the health effects of airborne contaminants in factory and urban air have come from epidemiology. Unfortunately, sometimes public agencies conduct "quick and dirty" studies that yield "quick and dirty" results that serve only to confound the issues rather than to provide answers.

The scenario in these cases often runs as follows: The public agency, usually at the behest of a legislative body, conducts a study in response to (or in anticipation of) a public outcry against the fouling of its air or water supply. The legislative body, not having an understanding of epidemiology, does not recognize the difficulties, complexities, and costs of such investigations. As a result, the request usually carries an unrealistic time limit of a few weeks or months, plus an inadequate budget. The public agency honors the request, usually because it is reluctant to tell the holder of the purse strings that its request is ill-conceived. The result is often a meaningless study that is of no value to the community because it neither finds statistically significant associations nor develops sufficient information to ease the worries of the community.

It is not possible to explain in one or two sentences why such requests cannot produce the information desired. Legislators are very busy and overworked people who, unfortunately, simply do not have time to become educated in such subjects as toxicology and epidemiology. Thus, a great deal of time and money are expended in producing meaningless data. The danger in such studies is that the public may be given a false sense of security, or an unjustified anxiety and concern, depending on the relationship of the findings to the facts of the situation.

Perhaps even more likely and more damaging is the fact that inconclusive studies often cause people to lose confidence in the public agencies that serve them. Quite often, the public has already decided that a local chemical plant is the cause of cancer cases in the vicinity or that groundwater contamination is the cause of birth defects in the neighborhood before a public agency undertakes an epidemiologic investigation. The public, unable to understand why its public officials cannot prove or disprove unequivocally the role of the chemical plant or the contaminated groundwater, decides that the public officials are incompetent and that its original assessment of blame is accurate.

THE PROXIMATE EVENT APPROACH IN ASSIGNING CAUSE

Cause–effect relationships are often obscure and difficult to ascertain, even in the face of strong associations. People not trained in the analytic techniques of epidemiology often fail to understand that a valid association between a cause and its effect cannot be made from a single case—a one-person epidemic—unless there are other independent data that support the association. As a result, there is a tendency for the public to use the proximate event approach in assigning causes for effects. For example, if a person suddenly becomes ill after eating lunch, or drinking a soft drink, he automatically blames the lunch or the soft drink, when the actual cause may very well have been something eaten the day or night before, or it may be due to the flu or some other infectious disease. Or a person may get the sniffles a few hours after visiting a friend at the hospital. The trip to the hospital, the place where everyone is sick, is blamed for the sniffles, when actually they are the result of a cold virus, with an incubation period of 7 to 11 days.

Occasionally, the proximate event approach is correct. If a person drinks several glasses of fruit punch or some other acid drink that was made and stored in a galvanized container, the chances are excellent that he will become very sick to his stomach very rapidly. The proximate event was the cause, and he would be correct in thinking so; sufficient zinc salts would have been dissolved from the galvanized coating by the acid liquid to make the punch emetic. However, the proof is not in the association between the punch and the illness but in the well-established fact that zinc salts are emetic and the demonstration of zinc salts in the punch.

Chemicals, particularly pesticides, often are innocent victims of the proximate event approach. The cat next door gives birth to a malformed kitten. The day before the lawn was sprayed with an herbicide; the herbicide is blamed for the malformation, when in actual fact the malformation would have had to have occurred at some time earlier in the kitten's fetal life. However, the proximate event approach may also be correct for pesticides. A person who sprays insecticides over large areas without using protective equipment and observing proper precautions may well show symptoms caused by the chemicals used.

There is no solution to the problem that misdiagnoses often result from attributing causes to proximate events. They are so easy and so apparently logical (and occasionally correct) that even physicians and scientists are sometimes guilty of using them, particularly when the scientific data are sparse. It is easier than searching further to determine if a proximate event is a probable or even a possible cause. Although little can be done to eliminate misuse of the proximate event approach, its existence and fallibility are worthy of a note of caution.

15

RISK

There is probably no human activity that does not carry with it some risk. However, it is only in recent years that risk has become something we think about on an almost daily basis. What is the risk of having a heart attack? What is the risk of getting AIDS? What is the risk of an earthquake or a tornado? What is the risk of a nuclear disaster? What is the risk that the greenhouse effect will occur? Our concerns run the gamut from very personal to global. What do we mean by risk and how do we evaluate it?

Risk refers to the chance that some unpleasantness, injury, loss, or other harm will befall us or someone or something we are concerned about. A consideration of risk, either intentionally or unknowingly, probably has always been part of human thought processes. Even small children rapidly learn the risks of arousing parental ire. Hardly a day goes by that we do not consider the risk presented by some activity, even if it is only as simple as not carrying an umbrella when the skies are threatening.

Risk has many facets. We hear of risk, risk assessment, perceived risk, acceptable risk, unacceptable risk, risk–benefit, risk communication, risk management, and so forth. What do these terms mean, where do they come from, and what is their importance to us? Public health statistics provided the earliest systematic basis for evaluating risks that affected groups of people.

PUBLIC HEALTH STATISTICS

A major goal of public health agencies is the prevention of disease. In order to prevent disease, the nature of diseases and their incidence in the population must be known. The bookkeeping of public health serves this mundane but essential role. Vital statistics, the record of births, deaths, and morbidity, are the product of public health bookkeeping. One use of vital statistics is to provide estimates of risk of occurrences of diseases.

The traditional method of expressing risk of disease has been based on historical information organized in the form of cause-specific death rates. These rates are calculated from the actual experience of a population group by counting the total number of people who died during a specified time period from a particular disease and dividing the deaths by the population at risk for that disease. The result is a number between zero and one. It expresses the fraction of the population that died from the disease. To make this fraction a whole number, public health statisticians usually multiply the fraction by 100,000. The result is the number of deaths per 100,000 population. For example, the rate of death from cancer of the respiratory system among white males living in the United States during 1950 was approximately 0.0002. In this example, the 0.0002 would be expressed as 20 per 100,000 population.

Public health statistics can be used to compare the relative impact of various diseases or examine the trend of diseases over a period of time. Using a specific disease as an example, in 1950, the death rate among white males from leukemia was approximately 7 per 100,000, or about one-third that from respiratory cancer. Statistics for 1980 show that the leukemia death rate has remained about the same from 1950 to 1980, while the death rate from respiratory cancer has almost tripled during this same period (Hodgson, T. A., Social and economic implications of cancer in the United States. In *Management of Assessed Risk for Carcinogens,* William J. Nicholson, ed., *Annals* **363**:189–204, 1981. New York: New York Academy of Sciences).

Such statistics can also be used to predict future risk presented by various causes of death. In making predictions, assumptions are made that "next year will be about the same as past years," or "next year will follow the trend established by past years." Depending on the nature of the disease, such forecasts can be quite accurate. A good example of this is actuarial forecasting done by insurance companies. Such forecasts are based on statistical calculations of life expectancy and the causes and rates of death according to population age groups. Causes may be age, accidents, or other risks covered by the insurance company. Risks are calculated for the purpose of determining what premiums the company should charge for insurance. In making their estimates, actuaries consider factors that modify risk, such as age, smoking practices, obesity, and past history of disease. The financial strength of the insurance industry over a period of many years is evidence that risks can be estimated with fair accuracy by using historical information on adverse outcomes and by continually adjusting these estimates as new information is available.

INHERENT RISK

The risk inherent in any situation or activity cannot be modified by whether the risk is considered acceptable or unacceptable, how great or small it is perceived to be, or even whether it is recognized as a risk. Risk can only be changed by altering the conditions that produce the risk. For example, the risk of developing cardiovascular disease from eating a diet high in saturated fats cannot be changed by accepting or rejecting the risk, by considering it to be important or of no consequence, or by not knowing it exists. The risk can be modified only by changing the diet or other factors responsible for the risk.

The actual chance that some harm or loss will occur and how great or small the inherent risk is cannot be known exactly, but in some cases it can be approximated. For example, no one knows the true risk of any one individual developing lung cancer from smoking, but a good estimate of what the chances might be can be made from examining the large body of data on the association between smoking and lung cancer. Risk estimates based on actuarial data can be quite accurate because they are based on records of adverse outcomes in large population groups. Further, the accuracy of the assumptions made for the estimates can be tested by how well they predict future occurrences.

On the other hand, many risks we face, particularly those associated with low-level exposure to environmental agents, cannot be estimated using traditional public health statistics. One reason is that morbidity and mortality statistics are based on medical diagnoses of causes of illness or death. The attending physician or autopsy surgeon can identify the immediate cause of death, such as bronchial cancer, leukemia, pancreatic cancer, or cardiovascular disease. At the present time, however, in many cases, medical science is unable to say what caused the cancer or other disease. This is especially true in the case of chemicals for which there are no known associations between exposure and some form of cancer.

Even with the very strong association between smoking and lung cancer, it can never be stated with certainty that a cancer in the lung of an individual smoker was caused by smoking. The reason is that although respiratory cancers, such as squamous cell cancer of the lung, are associated with smoking, they also occur in nonsmokers. If a squamous cell cancer occurs in a smoker, the chances are good that it was caused by smoking. However, it cannot be known that the cancer would not have occurred if the person had not smoked.

In the case of cigarette smoking, very large population studies have shown a clear association between smoking and increased rates of respiratory cancer. Studies with rodents have shown that smoke will cause higher rates of respiratory cancer. Some of the carcinogens in cigarette smoke have been identified and shown to cause cancer in test animals. Yet, as stated above, despite all of this evidence, it is impossible to prove that a particular respiratory cancer in an individual was caused by smoking. It is only possible to say that, based on population statistics and animal experimentation, the risk of respiratory cancer in that person was very much higher than it would have been had he been a nonsmoker.

With the exception of some very rare cancers that appear to be caused only by specific carcinogens, it is often impossible to determine the actual cause of any cancer in an individual. A similar situation exists for birth defects. Defects can be recorded, associations determined, and risks of occurrence estimated, but the specific cause in individual cases usually cannot be determined.

There are no statistics for many of the risks we face. Such is the case for the risk of cancer from environmental exposures to chemicals. There are no known cases of cancer (or birth defects) caused by exposure to trace quantities of any environmental chemical, natural or synthetic. As a general rule, medical diagnosis alone is unable to show a relationship between exposure to very small quantities of any chemical and cancer or birth defects. If there is good evidence from animal studies or occupational experience that some chemical is capable of causing cancer or birth defects, it may be assumed that a few cases could be caused by small exposures. However, at the present time there is no way of identifying those cases. Thus, estimates of risk of cancer or birth defects from exposure to trace amounts of a chemical cannot be based on a known incidence, nor can the accuracy or validity of the estimates be tested. In short, we can estimate the risk of occurrence of a particular kind of cancer, but we cannot accurately estimate the fraction, if any exists, of a particular cancer risk attributable to exposure to trace amounts of chemicals.

It is important to note that there are a few diseases caused by environmental agents that are directly diagnosable. Lead poisoning is a good example, even though the early symptoms of low-level exposure are vague and not particularly different from those of many minor illnesses. These symptoms include decreased physical fitness, tiredness, sleep disturbance, aching bones and muscles, abdominal pains, and constipation. Despite the vague symptoms, laboratory tests for levels of lead and certain biochemicals in blood can identify the cause of the illness and provide an estimate of the degree of poisoning.

Another example of an environmental agent that can be traced by the disease it produces is the organic chemical, vinyl chloride. Studies of workers exposed to very low levels of vinyl chloride have shown that this chemical causes a rare liver tumor known as angiosarcoma. This type of cancer is extremely rare and almost never found in people with no exposure to vinyl chloride.

RISK ASSESSMENT

When chronic toxicity testing became a common requirement a little more than 50 years ago, the emphasis was not on the risks associated with trace quantities of chemicals in foods but rather on what was a safe amount of exposure for the population. Tests were designed to determine no-effect levels in animals. Permissible levels for human exposure were set by applying margins of safety to no-effect levels determined in animal experimentation. Despite subsequent cries of outrage that so many carcinogens had been permitted to contaminate our food supply, the process worked well.

During the past decade a large number of chemicals have been retested using more sophisticated and more sensitive techniques. With the exception of a few chemicals that had a long history of use, such as some food color additives, retesting has not produced information that would require significant changes in regulatory procedures to protect public health. Despite greatly increased use of synthetic chemicals in food production and processing during the past 40 years, the general health of the nation has improved and life expectancy has gradually increased.

During the past two decades, people have become increasingly aware that some chemicals can cause cancer. Public fear and the resulting public demand for government regulation of chemical carcinogens created the need to estimate carcinogenic risk and set safe levels of exposure to such chemicals. There are two very serious obstacles to such a task. One, mentioned above, is the fact that there are no statistics. Excluding cancers from occupational exposures and a few rare forms of cancer known to be caused only by specific carcinogens, there are no documented cases of human cancer from exposure to trace quantities of chemical carcinogens. Despite the conviction that trace amounts of chemicals, such as pesticide residues, are causing cases of cancer, those cases cannot be identified. They cannot be identified because, if they are occurring, they are so few in number that they are hidden in the background incidence of cancer. If they cannot be identified, they cannot be counted.

The second obstacle to estimating carcinogenic risk and setting safe levels of exposure is the theory that there is no safe level of exposure to carcinogenic chemicals. This theory required that regulatory agencies reject the use of classic no-effect levels and thresholds for establishing permissible levels of exposure. The decision that the initiation of a cancer process is a chance (stochastic) event required a new approach for evaluating safety. The new approach was found in the procedure called risk assessment.

Risk assessment, as defined in this new approach, is the procedure by which an estimate of the chance that an untoward event will occur is made using elaborate statistical methodology. In cancer risk assessment, the untoward event is the occurrence of one or more cases of cancer as a result of exposure to a given quantity of carcinogen. Originally, the model used to estimate risk of cancer from chemical carcinogens was a one-hit (chemical bullet) model. The one-hit model is based on the premise that one molecule of a carcinogen can start a cancer process by striking a critical target in a cell, presumably a DNA molecule, and causing a mutation. The one-hit model for chemical carcinogenesis might be likened to a blindfolded shooter firing bullets at a moving target while blindfolded. What is the chance of hitting the target with one bullet? two bullets? and so on. The goal of the evaluation is to determine the number of bullets (carcinogenic molecules) that can be fired without exceeding an acceptable risk of hitting the target (DNA molecules).

All available scientific data on the subject demonstrate that chemical carcinogens do not act on a simple chance basis. A number of other controlling or modifying factors must be included in carcinogenic risk analysis. The addition of modifying factors greatly complicates the risk assessment process. Despite the complications, the simple one-hit model was expanded into a multistage model. Multistage models are based on the premise that, in addition to one hit by a molecule of carcinogen, one or more other conditions must exist, simultaneously or sequentially, before a cancer can be initiated. The one-hit model might be likened to the proposition that an automobile will start when the ignition is turned on. A multistage model would add that an automobile will start when the ignition is turned on *if* the battery is charged, and *if* the tank contains gasoline.

Numerous statistical models have been developed for the analysis of cancer risk from exposure to known or suspected human carcinogens. Different multistage models have been investigated by regulatory agencies because no one model seemed to satisfy all situations. Finally, a few have been accepted as being appropriate, but improvements and refinements continue to this date. The multistage models currently used in cancer risk assessment include the assumptions that a chemical that causes cancer in an animal study can cause cancer in humans, that human exposure to the carcinogen is daily for a lifetime of 70 years, and that one molecule of carcinogen is capable of causing cancer. Based on these assumptions, assessments are made to determine what level of carcinogenic risk is associated with various levels of human exposure to specific chemical carcinogens.

The people charged with protecting the public against dangerous exposures to carcinogens obviously must have some means for making estimates of what exposures are dangerous and what exposures would be virtually safe. However, in the process of estimating risk, mathematical models and formulas should be an adjunct to, and not a substitute for, scientific judgment. In addition, regulatory agencies must be free from special-interest pressures if the standards they promulgate are to be based on concern for the public good, not political expediency.

A review of the megamouse study (see Chapter 10) by the Society of Toxicology (SOT) includes a concise, clear statement that addresses the issue of cancer risk assessment:

> The SOT Task Force recognizes the need for establishing acceptable exposure levels and the significant need for societal (regulatory) understanding of the effects of chronic low level exposure to potential carcinogenic materials. The Task Force further acknowledges that the determination of the acceptability of risk is a societal (regulatory) decision. However, the Task Force strongly asserts that the evaluation of toxicological responses (carcinogenic or otherwise) and the estimation of risk to a given exposure is a scientific endeavor and must be conducted free and separate from regulatory considerations. The scientific estimate of risk must use appropriate methods (models) to obtain "best" estimates for risk with levels of confidence clearly stated. The use of the most conservative methods (models) for estimating risk can be both scientifically inappropriate and misleading to those charged with the responsibility of setting levels of acceptable risk. When "best estimates" models are used which incorporate time to tumor data into risk assessment as opposed to only adjusting for time, the ED_{01} Study demonstrates that linear quantal models, i.e., non-threshold models, do not fit the data and non-linear models which often suggest practical thresholds provide a better expression of observed responses. (Reexamination of the ED_{01} study, *Fundamental and Applied Toxicology* 1(1):29, 1981).

The literature is replete with papers describing the various models used for carcinogenic risk assessment. A journal entitled *Risk Analysis,* the official journal for the Society for Risk Analysis, published by Plenum Press, had its debut in March 1981 in response to the increasing need for communication among scientists and regulators. This journal would be an excellent source for anyone interested in more information on the subject of risk. *Risk Analysis* presents papers dealing with all aspects of risk, not just risk assessment procedures.

A fair amount of knowledge of statistical methodology is necessary for an understanding of the models used in risk assessment. People without such knowledge, but who want more information on risk assessment, will find the review of the risk assessment process, its history, its definitions, and its methods written by L. D. Hopper and F. W. Oehme for *Veterinary and Human Toxicology* (31(6):543–554, 1989) a valuable introduction to the subject.

PERCEIVED RISK

How people perceive risk has been the subject of many social and psychological studies because of its importance to decisions made to control risks. Legislators and regulators can obtain assessments of risk from scientists and statisticians. However, since the public often perceives a risk differently from the way it is described by the risk assessment process, legislators must also know how the public views the same risk and the reasons for the perception.

Decisions by local government agencies are more often based on the public's perception of risk than on assessments made by scientists. A major goal of politicians is to be reelected, a goal that will not be achieved if they antagonize the electorate. Since local officials are closer to their constituents than state and federal officials, they are more vulnerable to public displeasure. For example, no matter how small a risk of reduced air quality is posed by a waste-to-energy conversion plant, and despite great need for management of household waste, some people would oppose having such a facility in their community because they consider the risk associated with incineration unacceptable, particularly in their own neighborhoods. The decision by local officials about building such a facility would depend largely on the strength of the opposition rather than on scientific or statistical risk assessment.

Risk perception is a very personal matter, and a very complex one. Just as no two people have the exact same fingerprints, so there are probably no two people who have the exact same perceptions of all possible risks. Risks based on the same value system may be viewed similarly by people who share the same system, but many risks are not linked. For example, some people are terrified of flying, and others enjoy it immensely without fear. Yet some people from both groups share a perception that smoking cigarettes is a very dangerous activity. Others from both groups enjoy smoking and consider that the surgeon general's warnings are considerably overexaggerated. The risks associated with flying and with smoking, like so many other risks, are not coupled; they are viewed independently.

A brief mention of some of the factors that influence perception of risk, hopefully, will be of value to an understanding of one's own perceptions, particularly those relating to risks associated with chemicals. The closer the public's perception of a specific risk agrees with the risk determined by an objective scientific and statistical risk assessment process, the greater the chances that regulatory decisions will be based on knowledge rather than on emotion, and that good and lasting benefit will accrue to society from the controls imposed. When all facets of society, industry, government, and the public agree on the magnitude of a risk, political decisions made to control the risk will be more generally acceptable and cooperation with regulations will be more easy to obtain.

Education is an obvious factor in risk perception. Education has a number of definitions. It may refer to the kind of education, the level of education, or the source of education. As a general rule, people educated in one discipline see the risks associated with the technologies developed from their disciplines much differently than people educated in other fields. Recent concerns about genetic engineering provide an example of difference in perception of risk depending on kind of education. Microbiologists view the risk to public or environmental health from the manipulation of genetic composition of microorganisms differently than people educated in other disciplines. They know the processes, the significance of the alterations, the controls employed, and so forth.

People who have less than a college education perceive risks differently than people who have had a higher education. The differences cannot be attributed to lesser intelligence. Many people with average or above intelligence do not go beyond high school for a number of reasons. The reasons include lack of finances or financial support, lack of interest in academic subjects, family or peer pressures, and so forth. Blue-collar workers often see the risks associated with their occupations as being less than indicated by statistics on occupational illness and injury.

A major source of education for a majority of people is the news media—television, radio, and the print media. Television and radio commentators seldom have the luxury of delving into any news story with the breadth and depth required to provide the viewer with sufficient facts to make informed decisions. Journalists who write for newspapers and magazines do have more time to ascertain facts and more space to present a balanced story. Some may see themselves merely as reporters, but they are, in fact, educators.

Education is only one of many factors that influence perceptions of risk. Other factors can be of equal or greater importance, depending on the nature of the hazard and the risk involved. These include such diverse conditions as social status, economic status, age, sex, sexual orientation, national origin, place of residence, racial and cultural background, religious orientation, and opinions of friends and relatives.

Risk perception has been the subject of numerous studies by social scientists. Paul Slovic, William Lowrance, and Aaron Wildavsky are among the many who have written interesting and informative books on the subject (see the Suggested Reading section). The journal *Risk Analysis* is also a good source for further reading.

ACCEPTABLE RISK

The acceptability of a risk may be viewed from two levels, societal and personal. On the societal level, the process is generally as follows: The responsible governmental agency holds public hearings to obtain testimony from scientists and members of the public. When all information is gathered, the agency quantifies the risk using statistical methods referred to in the section on risk assessment, above.

After the risk has been quantified, a further policy decision must be made as to how much risk is acceptable. In the case of cancer risk assessments, regulatory agencies are faced with the weighty responsibility of having to decide how many cancer cases due to a carcinogen would be acceptable. Government officials, acting for society, have decided that one excess cancer in a population of a million constitutes an acceptable risk.

There are a number of problems associated with assigning a specific figure to the number of cases of cancer considered acceptable. It gives the false impression that the figure is a matter of scientific fact rather than a statistically derived estimate. It delivers the erroneous message that one in a million people, no more, no less, will actually develop cancer from exposure to the chemical in question. It misleads the public into believing that one extra case of cancer in a population of a million people actually could be measured and the cause could be identified. Finally, it frightens some people who fear that they or one of their loved ones may become that one unfortunate soul in a million. They wonder why their government would consider that *any* extra cases of cancer are acceptable. Stevie O. Daniels, former executive editor of *Organic Gardening,* articulated these concerns in her March 1989 editorial:

> The EPA defines negligible risk for adults as a one-in-a-million chance of getting cancer from a particular residue in a lifetime. . . . That means roughly 231 people will develop cancer. . . . What kind of a world do we have if we accept the incidence of cancer in one in every million people?

On a personal level, the determination that a risk is acceptable (or unacceptable) is quite a different matter. Often, people reject societal decisions concerning acceptability. The organic food movement is a case in point.

People who purchase only produce grown without the use of pesticides reject the societal decision that the risk of cancer from exposure to trace quantities of pesticides is negligible (acceptable).

Personal decisions concerning the acceptability of risk are not based on statistical models. Rather, they are based on how the risks are perceived. Whether the risks are familiar or foreign, voluntary or involuntary, result in a mild inconvenience or a disaster, and so forth, all play a role in their acceptance or rejection by individuals.

RISK-BENEFIT AND COST-BENEFIT

Risk-benefit and cost-benefit might be likened to two sides of a coin. The former balances the risk involved in some action or event against the benefit derived. The latter examines the cost of some action, such as reduction of a risk, in relation to the benefit achieved.

Almost every risk can be subjected to evaluation of benefits and costs from both personal and societal perspectives. For example, the risk of not wearing a helmet when riding a motorcycle is suffering a massive head injury in case of an accident. For the individual, the benefit of not wearing a helmet might be the pleasure of feeling the wind blow through his hair. Some cyclists feel the benefit is worth the risk. For society there is no benefit. In fact, society has enacted laws requiring the wearing of helmets because it has decided that, in the absence of benefit, the cost of caring for people permanently disabled with massive head injuries is unacceptable.

Chlorination of drinking water is another example in which there are individual and societal risk-benefit and cost-benefit considerations. Public drinking water supplies are chlorinated to kill pathogens that cause serious illness or death. The risk from chlorination is the production of trace amounts of chemicals suspected of causing cancer, such as chloroform. The risk of not chlorinating public water supplies is the occurrence of mass outbreaks of water-borne diseases. For society, the former risk is negligible whereas the latter risk is unacceptable. The benefit of chlorination is considered by society to be more than worth the cost. Most people probably give little thought to the matter. However, for a few individuals, the risk of exposure to trace quantities of carcinogens, no matter how slight, is unacceptable. For them, avoiding the perceived risk is worth the cost of bottled water.

The regulation of chemicals, particularly chemicals that cause or are suspected of causing cancer, is the result of public demand for such controls. Few would dispute the need for government regulation of hazardous chemicals to protect the public health from exposure to toxic and carcinogenic chemicals in workplaces, homes, and general environment. In addition to need for regulation, legislators also recognize that risks, benefits, and costs must all be taken into consideration when setting standards for chemical exposures. The reason is the very practical one that regulation of chemicals costs money, taxpayers' money, and the legislators are responsible for obtaining the funds required from the taxpayers. Unfortunately, people usually do not consider the cost of regulation and are not as involved as they should be in demanding rigorous risk-cost-benefit evaluations from their government officials.

The regulation of chemical carcinogens is a case in point. The cancer risk models used by regulatory agencies assume that one molecule of a carcinogen is capable of initiating a cancer process, that exposure to the carcinogen is a lifetime exposure (daily exposure for 70 years), and that data obtained from animal carcinogenicity studies are directly translatable to humans. Cancer risk estimates derived from these models are very conservative because of the nature of the assumptions upon which they are based. It is usual and appropriate for public officials to err on the side of safety in matters relating to public and environmental health, if they are going to err at all. Regulatory agencies acknowledge that the cancer risk estimates that are currently being used for regulatory purposes have a large error on the side of safety. Thus, if the assumptions used by regulatory agencies are incorrect, the errors can only result in excess safety for the public, not less safety. If regulations are based on risk assessments that are in error by several orders of magnitude, the benefits to society could well be negligible or nonexistent and the costs to taxpayers could be overburdening.

Society has the right to decide on the level of safety it wants. It also has a right to know the cost increments for each increase in degree of safety so it can decide if the benefits are worth the cost. However, it must be kept in mind that risk, benefit, and cost evaluations are only proper when the risk takers, benefit receivers, and pocketbooks are the same or equivalent. For example, assume that a person decides to paint his house himself in order to save money. One risk he faces is injury from falling off the ladder. The benefit is that he saves money. The risk and benefit are equitable—he takes the risk and he reaps the benefit. On the other hand, assume a factory decides to speed up an assembly line to increase profits. One risk is that a worker may suffer injury from the more rapidly running machinery. The benefit is increased profits for the company. In such a situation the risk and benefit are not equitable—the worker takes the risk and the company receives the benefit.

RISK COMMUNICATION

Risk communication embraces the very delicate task of explaining all aspects of risks to the public. The average citizen is perfectly capable of understanding complex subjects that are of interest or importance to him. Unfortunately, government, industry, and academic scientists are not always capable of making complex subjects understandable. Scientists have much to learn about communication with the public. They must recognize not only that the nomenclatures of their sciences are not familiar to the average person but also that their nomenclature can be translated into common terms.

People also have a responsibility in the communication process. They must appreciate that most scientists have little experience in communicating with the public and that many are intimidated by the public. People should attempt to learn the meaning of some scientific words and terms to help them better evaluate conflicting opinions about risks. Some civic groups, such as the League of Women Voters, provide forums for interaction between scientists and the community because they recognize the need for public understanding of environmental issues. Industry, consumer groups, government, environmental groups, and civic groups must learn to communicate with each other—to discuss openly and rationally the pros and cons of arguments relating to environmental matters.

Risk communication can carry with it its own special kind of risk for scientists who attempt to explain their sciences to the public objectively and in nontechnical terms. In doing so they face the risk of being labeled as apologists by one side or the other of an issue, or perhaps by both. This is particularly true in the fields of toxicology and carcinogenesis. Scientists who attempt to put the risks from exposure to trace quantities of synthetic chemicals into a proper perspective are met with derision by environmental partisans. As a result, some scientists are hesitant to take part in public debates.

Journalists form one of the most important communication links between science and the public. Much of what the public knows about the risks and benefits of science and technology is obtained from newspaper and magazine articles. Even scientists themselves gain some of their knowledge of other sciences from the same source as the general public—the news media. The importance of journalists in informing the public and, as a consequence, shaping public policy cannot be overstated. Victor Cohen, a senior writer for the *Washington Post,* describes the journalist's position in *Health Risks and the Press* (see the Selected Reading section, Moore, M., ed.):

Whether we like it or not, we journalists have become gatekeepers. In some measure, our choices of what will be reported, and how the data will be reported, set the national agenda vis-a-vis health risks. In a sense, we have become part of the regulatory machinery. . . . The very way we report a situation can affect the outcome. If we ignore a bad situation or write a "no danger" piece, the public may suffer. If we write "danger" the public may quake.

Journalists are often blamed for the public's misunderstanding or lack of appreciation of the safety or danger of some technology when circumstances beyond their control may really be at fault. Journalists can only communicate information given to them by their sources. Sources may not express themselves clearly, they may exaggerate, or they may voice conflicting opinions; experts of seemingly equal repute often disagree with each other. In addition, there are the ever-present time and space constraints that limit a journalist's ability to explain the nuances of a story. Time and space constraints are probably also responsible for some instances in which scientists feel they have been misquoted or their words have been taken out of context. And finally, the public's penchant for stories that are brief with dramatic or frightening headlines guides editors who are the final authority about what gets into print.

The majority of professional journalists are truly interested in serving their communities through the media. Those who attempt to explain both sides of issues so that readers can form their own opinions perform a valuable public service. Further, competent journalists will investigate the competence and biases of their sources so they can better evaluate the information they receive. Journalists who permit their personal biases to influence the content of their news stories can do a great deal of damage, particularly if they write well and interestingly. Unfortunately, some journalists who let their biases show in their reporting do not recognize their own failing. They may feel they are performing a public service, but if they misinform and mislead the public, deliberately or inadvertently, they are subverting an informed electorate. People who have access to reports of journalists who present all sides of an issue, particularly science issues, free of editorializing, are truly fortunate!

The popular press is also an important avenue for risk communication. A number of scientists, through lectures, essays, and books, have become as influential as journalists in forming public opinion. Some of these scientists describe the risks to society presented by science and technology in general, and the petrochemical industry in particular. Some have publicly aligned themselves with one or more environmental or social causes that they support with great fervor. Other scientists who are unaligned with any pro- or antichemical movement attempt to provide the public with a balanced perspective of the risks associated with chemicals in the environment. In the latter group, there are a few who attempt to counter the biases that feed poison paranoia by examining the arguments, actions, and motives of the antiscience and antitechnology movements. There are many books and articles, such as those by Vincent Covello or Paul Slovic (see the Suggested Reading section), describing all aspects of the subject of risks presented by natural and synthetic chemicals available to people who are interested in studying all sides of the issues.

Unfortunately, there are some people whose minds are closed to any idea contrary to their convictions, regardless of whether they are convinced that some technology is perfect and has no drawbacks, or that some technology is all bad and has no virtues. There can be no communication with people with closed minds. Fortunately, they represent a minority of the public. The majority of people do have open minds and are willing to listen to opposing views. In scientific matters, as in every other facet of human endeavor and interaction, there is no substitute for communication.

RISK MANAGEMENT

Risk management is the control of risk by eliminating or modifying the conditions that produce the risk. People practice risk management in all aspects of daily life, often without realizing it. The parent who stores medicines and household chemicals out of a child's reach is practicing risk management. The driver who fastens his seat belt is practicing risk management. The hobbyist who provides good ventilation in the area where solvents are used is practicing risk management. The gardener who puts on protective clothing before spraying pesticides is practicing risk management. The chemist who puts on safety glasses before entering the laboratory is practicing risk management.

Governments practice risk management by passing rules and regulations that specify procedures for controlling risks and penalties for disregard of the procedures. The risks that governments manage are those that affect the public in general or specific groups of people. Businesses, industries, and public agencies become the risk managers by complying with the rules and regulations. However, before government can manage a risk, the risk must be recognized, described, and its importance to society must be evaluated. This process requires time, money, and considerable effort in laboratory and field research. The public, not recognizing the difficulties involved in the process, often becomes impatient with regulatory agencies for not acting rapidly enough to protect it. The risk management agency that has suffered the greatest amount of criticism is the EPA.

The EPA was created in 1970 with the broad and almost unmanageable mandate to protect both public health and environmental health. It was created in response to public concerns that pesticides were destroying the habitat and the inhabitants of the planet. In its more than 20 years of existence, EPA has done an amazingly good job despite the tremendous difficulties under which it has had to operate. It has restored the ecological balance in some locations that formerly had been sites of major water or air pollution and has prevented further deterioration in other areas. Unfortunately, EPA's public image has never equaled its accomplishments. A brief review of the evolution of public and political concerns that led to the creation of EPA is given by Jack Lewis in "Looking Backward: A Historical Perspective on Environmental Regulations" (*EPA Journal,* p. 26, March 1988).

Risk management is most effective when combined with risk communication. Local industries that fail to communicate their activities to concerned citizens may face community antipathy and opposition, and perhaps even restrictive legislation by local governments. Companies that explain their problems and listen to the concerns of their neighbors in open two-way communication are those most likely to achieve successful risk management programs. Programs of risk communication and risk management that involve the community take considerable top management and staff time and can add to costs, but the benefits of community understanding and cooperation could be more than worth the expenditure. Companies that are responsible citizens and the communities in which they reside both benefit from the relationship.

16

PUBLIC DISTRUST
OF SCIENCE

Despite the fact that public opinion polls give science high marks as a respected profession, the past few decades have witnessed an erosion of public confidence in scientists, their accomplishments, and the validity of their judgments. One of my favorite cartoonists epitomized this public attitude in a cartoon strip showing Señors Dog and Owl lying on their backs on a grassy slope, gazing lazily at the sky. Señor Owl says, "Is this the latter part of June? 85 tons of skylab will drop on us any day now! Scientists are a menace!" Señor Dog replies, "Whoa, owl! Don't forget, after all, scientists brought us double knits, plastics, pesticides, preservatives, automobiles, asbestos, amplified music, television, nuclear fission," which leads to Señor Owl's punch line, "I repeat! Scientists are a menace!" (Gus Arriola, Gordo. *San Francisco Chronicle,* June 19, 1979).

Public distrust is directed primarily against those sciences and attendant technologies that are viewed as sources of some manner of threat to human or environmental health and well-being. Many excellent, thoughtful essays on the subject of public doubts about science have appeared in scientific periodicals. The subject is very complex and of concern to many physical, biological, and social scientists. A great deal of profound thought on the part of some of the best minds in their respective fields has been devoted to the problem. Thus, it would be presumptuous to consider that the issue could be discussed adequately within the pages of this chapter. Rather, the purpose of this chapter is to examine some of the probable reasons for public skepticism relating to issues within the field of toxicology. Hopefully, such an examination will help replace distrust with open-mindedness, or at least with an attitude of tolerance. Public distrust of science benefits no one, least of all the public who is the most affected by the applications of scientific discoveries.

DILEMMAS

One reason for public distrust or confusion may be the abundance of contradictory information that is presented in the news media on an almost daily basis. The conflict between the benefits derived from chemicals and the hazards of their use will never cease to provide society and individuals with numerous dilemmas to resolve. Medical science has found that diets low in cholesterol carry a several-fold increase in risk of cancer of the colon than diets high in cholesterol. but diets high in cholesterol are implicated in a much greater risk of cardiovascular disease. Nitrites in cured meats are required to prevent the growth of the organisms responsible for deadly botulism. But epidemiologic evidence indicates that diets high in nitrites carry a greater risk of stomach cancer. The various birth control pill formulations have proven to be very effective in preventing the tragedy of unwanted pregnancy. But medical science warns of the risk of potentially serious adverse reactions with protracted use of some birth control pills. Women at the age of menopause who take estrogen compounds to relieve the distressing symptoms that occur with the change of life are warned that estrogens increase their risk of uterine cancer. But estrogens also are protective against osteoporosis, a major cause of life-threatening fractures of the hip, which are so common to postmenopausal women. Examples of dilemmas are endless. What information should a person seek?

The first question to ask is, Is there a substitute chemical or a different method for achieving the same end? The next question is, What are the risks versus the benefits? Judicious questioning of medical societies, public health departments, federal agencies such as EPA and FDA, private agencies such as the American Cancer Society or the American Heart Association, educational institutions, libraries, or any other appropriate individuals or groups, will help provide the data necessary to evaluate the problem. However, it must be kept in mind that a few agencies, both public and private, have actually become advocates for one side or another of a particular issue despite the fact that they maintain a facade of objectivity. Therefore, one should obtain as much information as possible from as many different sources as possible. From that point on, it is an individual decision to be made or perhaps a matter to be lobbied with a legislator.

It has become common in recent years for environmental or consumer groups to demand that chemicals they consider detrimental to their special interests be banned. The banning of chemicals is a simplistic solution to a very complex problem and often produces greater problems than those sought to be remedied by the ban. In some cases it requires the elimination of a chemical whose toxic properties and hazards are quite well known, and substitution with a chemical or chemicals about which there is much less information. The banning of chemicals denies man's ingenuity to develop methods of use that will be protective of the health of the public and of the environment, and it denies society the benefits they contribute. Proponents of bans either do not accept that the chemicals in question can be used safely or contend that the malevolence and greed of industry will not permit safe use.

Like so many other issues related to the toxicity of chemicals, politics and special interest pressures override and obscure the true nature of toxic hazards. Actually, there is no chemical so toxic that it cannot be worked with safely, even if it requires the extremes of remote control operation or totally enclosed space suits with clean-air supply. The aerospace industry has learned full well to work with some of the most toxic of materials. Such highly toxic chemicals seldom are brought into ordinary channels of industry and commerce and so are never contacted by the general public. Like so many other matters relating to use of chemicals, the issue of chemical bans is one that effects the entire population and so must be settled according to the wishes of society, it is hoped an informed society.

TRANS-SCIENCE

Fundamental to the question of why the public has come to distrust the sciences that deal with human and environmental health is the uncertain nature of those sciences. Unlike physics and mathematics, the health sciences cannot provide us with absolute or, in some instances, even reasonably certain answers. People do not question whether an apple will fall to the ground rather than fly skyward when it detaches from its tree. People do not question whether a half of a pie is less than its whole or that the whole pie is equal to all of the pieces cut from it. But people are skeptical about data concerning the health risks, or lack thereof, posed by exposure to synthetic chemicals. Why? Alvin M. Weinberg's introduction of the concept of trans-science provides a proper backdrop for an examination of this question and whole issue of public skepticism or frank distrust of science.

The term *trans-science* was proposed by Dr. Weinberg to describe the limitations of scientific methodology in providing data required by some issues of concern to society (Science and trans-science. *Minerva* 10(2):209–222, 1972). In his discussion of the relation between scientific knowledge and societal decisions he notes,

> Many of the issues which arise in the course of the interaction between science or technology and society . . . hang on the answers

to questions which can be asked of science and yet *which cannot be answered by science*. I propose the term *trans-scientific* for these questions since, though they are, epistemologically speaking, questions of fact and can be stated in the language of science, they are unanswerable by science; they transcend science.

Dr. Weinberg cites three causes for the inability of science to answer trans-scientific questions:

[1] Science is inadequate simply because to get answers would be impractically expensive. . . . [2] Science is inadequate because the subject-matter is too variable to allow rationalisation according to the strict scientific canons established within the natural sciences. . . . [3] Science is inadequate simply because the issues themselves involve moral and esthetic judgments: they deal not with what is true but rather with what is valuable.

Many trans-scientific questions asked of toxicology can be placed in the first category, which, for our purposes, will also include questions that science does not yet have sufficient knowledge or techniques to answer.

The questions uppermost in the minds of individuals relate to whether or not exposure to some chemical or chemicals will be harmful to their health or that of their loved ones. Often these are the very questions that toxicology cannot answer with a definite "yes" or "no." Science has no way of knowing the exact biochemical makeup of any individual person or exactly what quantity of chemical would be just below that person's threshold for the most subtle adverse effect of which the chemical is capable. An answer based on judgment *can* be given, but science does not as yet (and may very well never) have the methodology to respond to these concerns with direct experimental evidence. However, answers based on scientific judgment, no matter how well founded, are often rejected because people want absolute answers, not best guesses, to questions concerning their health. The issue is further confused because best guesses tend to vary among scientists. The validity of a guess depends on the expertise of the scientist who offers it.

The questions uppermost in the minds of legislators and regulatory officials relate to the nature and incidence of adverse effects that might result from exposure of large populations of humans to very small quantities of environmental contaminants. Science does not have the resources—money, trained personnel, laboratory facilities, experimental animals—to provide such information for even a few, much less all, of the many chemicals we may encounter in our daily lives. Legislators and regulatory officials, like their constituents, want absolute answers. They fail to understand why definitive experimental studies cannot be conducted to provide such answers.

Dr. Weinberg's example illustrating the impracticability of such experimental studies deals with radiation effects, but it could as well apply to any chemical exposure:

> Let us consider the biological effects of low-level radiation insults to the environment, in particular the genetic effects of low levels of radiation on mice. Experiments performed at high radiation levels show that the dose required to double the spontaneous mutation rate in mice is 30 roentgens of X-rays. Thus, if the genetic response to X-radiation is linear, then a dose of 150 millirems would increase the spontaneous mutation rate in mice by 1/2 per cent. . . . Now, to determine at the 95 per cent. confidence level by direct experiment whether 150 millirems will increase the mutation rate by 1/2 per cent. requires about 8,000,000,000 mice! Of course this number falls if one reduces the confidence level: at 60 per cent. confidence level, the number is 195,000,000. Nevertheless, the number is so staggeringly large that, as a practical matter, the question is unanswerable by direct scientific investigation.

Dr. Weinberg's example tells us that, in essence, an effect that has a very low incidence of occurrence would almost certainly not be seen in an experiment using only a few animals. A study using 10 animals will not reveal an effect that occurs in only 1 out of 100,000 animals. In order to demonstrate such an effect, many times 100,000 animals would be required. Experiments of that magnitude are beyond the capability of existing resources and so are in the realm of trans-science.

PUBLIC EXPECTATIONS EXCEED SCIENCE'S CAPABILITIES

Public skepticism is a natural consequence of the fact that the public expects more of scientists than they are able to provide. People not only want absolute answers, as described above, but often they want answers that are in agreement with what they believe. For example, when a local dump or hazardous waste site is suspected of causing an excess number of birth defects, local officials or legislators often demand to know why the local health agency does not "just go in there and find out," not realizing the great difficulty of such a task. Or, when the public wants to know if local industrial air pollutants are causing lung cancer, they do not understand why an immediate answer cannot be given.

All too often, in such cases, the public has already decided that the dump or waste site is causing birth defects, or that industry effluents are causing lung cancer. Thus, if a biostatistical study of the pollution sources and rates of disease in the area indicates that there is no association between the pollution and the adverse effects, some people reject the report claiming that a more competent study would show an association or that industry interests biased the results. Public skepticism is often intensified in such circumstances because of qualifications appended to study reports. Scientists who conduct biostatistical studies usually state, rightfully so, that their findings cannot be considered conclusive because of weaknesses and statistical uncertainty inherent in such studies.

Health bureaucracies, unfortunately, are often unable to cope with public skepticism. Public meetings convened in response to public concern about some local environmental issue are often difficult for all concerned. In some instances, health officials appear dictatorial or paternalistic because, even though they have the knowledge and expertise, the kinds of scientific studies required to respond to public concerns and gain public confidence are not feasible. In other instances, the health officials, though well-motivated, do not have the knowledge or expertise and, thus, appear to the public as incompetent bureaucrats.

Occasionally, the health officials themselves privately believe that there is a cause–effect relationship even though the data are inadequate to show an association. Thus, they are not convincing. They use phrases such as, "The data are provocative, but we can't say there's a relationship." Such equivocal statements serve to stimulate further skepticism and public distrust. Health agencies that are successful in gaining public confidence and cooperation are those that not only explain and educate but also involve members of the public in investigations and evaluations of the problems at hand. People who are given such a role, along with a voice in the decision-making process, seldom throw tomatoes in public meetings.

THE INABILITY TO PROVE A NEGATIVE

Dr. Weinberg, in his article on trans-science, mentions another point that is important to an understanding of the limitations of toxicological science and the resulting public distrust:

> No matter how large the experiment, even if *no* effect is observed, one can still only say there is a certain probability that there is in fact no effect. One can never, with any finite experiment, prove that any environmental factor is totally harmless. This elementary point has unfortunately been lost in much of the public discussion of environmental hazards.

This brings us to one of the most frustrating matters with which toxicologists and health professionals must cope, namely, proving absolute safety of exposure to chemicals. It is most natural for people to demand assurance that the chemical exposures they experience are absolutely safe, and it is very difficult for them to grasp the fact that this is an assurance that no one is capable of giving. Absolute safety is the complete absence of harm—the nonexistence of harm. How does anyone prove the nonexistence of anything?

Negative toxicologic data always prompt further questions. If a toxicity experiment shows a certain level of exposure to be a no-effect level, the question can be asked, "What if more animals had been used?" If more animals yield the same result: "What if the study had been continued through one or two generations?" If a two-generation study yields the same results, then: "What might happen after 5 generations?" "10 generations?" "20 generations?" There is no such thing as a diminishing supply of questions. There is always one more unanswered one.

There is also no such thing as a diminishing supply of skepticism. A number of years ago, during a panel discussion on the use of herbicides in forestry, a man in the audience stated that the concept of the no-effect level was just not logical. He stated that there must be a chemical somewhere in the world that would be harmful no matter how small a dose was given. This seems to be a very rational observation. It is not unreasonable for people to consider that some chemicals may be harmful no matter how small the dose. However, there is no way to prove that such a chemical does or does not exist. For any chemical that does produce adverse effects down to the smallest dose that can be administered practically, there is no direct way to prove that some much smaller dose would be harmless. By the same token, there is also no way to prove that those smaller doses would be harmful. People who hold opposing views of what the correct answer is to a trans-scientific question are on equal ground.

The fact that toxicology cannot provide absolute answers to many of the questions that are of great concern to people should not be cause for alarm. Toxicologists *can* make judgments about the possibilities and probabilities of harm resulting from exposure to chemicals. These judgments are based on scientific data obtained from chronic toxicity testing, knowledge of the behavior of the chemical in animal systems, and application of appropriate margins of safety.

ALL SCIENTISTS KNOW ALL SCIENCE? (DOCTORS, LAWYERS, AND HIGH PRIESTS)

Another factor that contributes to public mistrust or skepticism of scientists who deal with toxicologic questions stems from the perception that there is a fair amount of disagreement among experts. These disagreements cover a variety of subjects such as the toxic or carcinogenic potency of specific chemicals, the nature or degree of hazard posed by certain chemical applications or exposures, the adequacy of testing procedures, the interpretation of data, and so forth. Such disagreement among experts could not fail to shake the faith even of people educated in the sciences if they did not understand the roots of the disagreement. Why do the experts disagree? There probably are as many reasons as there are experts.

Questions that are in the realm of trans-science provide a fertile ground for disagreement in any field of scientific endeavor. A further contribution to disagreements among scientists on toxicologic matters is that scientists are not all operating from the same base of knowledge. The public perception seems to be that scientists are all of one kind, and that they all are expert in all matters scientific—a scientist is a scientist. Nothing could be further from the truth.

People do not have difficulty with the fact that there are many scientific disciplines. They recognize that science is divided into major categories, such as biology, chemistry, physics, geology, and astronomy, and that each major category contains many subdivisions. However, when it comes to the expertise of individual scientists, people do not seem to discern that an authority in one field is not, of necessity, an authority in all of the others. In fact, quite often an expert in one scientific field is not even expert in another that is closely related in subject matter. Despite the fact that the fund of scientific knowledge has become so great that no one person can master more than a fraction of it, a person has only to proclaim himself a scientist, and people will automatically accept him as a possessor of all knowledge.

There are many scientific disciplines that deal with toxic effects of chemicals. For example, biochemists study the pathways of metabolism of toxicants, molecular biologists study adverse effects at the molecular level, microbiologists study adverse effects in single-celled organisms, plant pathologists study toxic effects in plants, environmental scientists study the impact of chemicals on the environment, pharmacologists and toxicologists study adverse effects in animals and humans, and, in the practical application of medical science, veterinarians and physicians diagnose and treat the adverse effects of toxicants in animals and humans, respectively. Thus, there are many scientists from a host of scientific disciplines who, along with toxicologists, expound on the toxic properties of chemicals. Molecular biochemists and microbiologists, for example, may well have great expertise in the effects of chemicals at the molecular or cellular levels, but unless they understand the principles that govern the more complex organisms, such as humans, they have no basis for making judgments, much less public statements, on the significance for humans of the effects they find in their test systems.

Criticism of individual scientists who make pronouncements on the toxicity of chemicals for humans without being qualified to do so should not be taken as demeaning the contributions of other life sciences to the fields of pharmacology and toxicology. In fact, the ultimate understanding of the effects of chemicals, both beneficial and harmful, requires knowledge from all of these allied disciplines. Toxicologists must know how chemicals behave at the molecular and cellular levels, what biochemical reactions they undergo, how they are influenced by various nutrients and nutritional states, and so forth, if the nature of the toxicity of chemicals is to be fully understood. For this knowledge they are dependent on the other biological sciences.

Physicians comprise another professional group whose dictums carry great weight with the public. There is a small fraction of the medical community whose livelihood is dependent on public fear of environmental chemicals. Practitioners in this group misuse accepted analytical, diagnostic, and treatment methods, such as hair analysis and EDTA chelation therapy, to diagnose and treat a wide variety of medical ailments they claim are due to exposure to environmental chemicals. Even excluding these practitioners, who are on the fringe of or outside ethical medicine, there still exists in the medical community some lack of understanding of adverse effects of chemicals.

Medical education covers such a tremendously wide range and quantity of information necessary to the diagnosis and treatment of disease that ancillary subjects such as toxicology and occupational medicine are given only superficial consideration. As a result, there are a few physicians who fail to recognize the universality of pharmacologic principles and believe that the laws of pharmacology apply only to drugs. They accept the no-effect concept for drugs, but not for food additives, pesticide residues, and so on. Their incomplete knowledge of toxicologic principles gives them little basis for making judgments about the significance of most chronic exposures for humans. Many patients find it difficult to accept that their physicians are not necessarily expert in toxicology.

Criticism of the few physicians who make public statements about the toxicity of chemicals, for which there are no bases in fact, should not detract from the very valuable contributions to the science of toxicology by physicians who are, in fact, toxicologists. It should also not be taken as a deprecation of the medical profession. Medical practice is a very demanding profession that requires a dedication and sacrifice that the majority of people would not suffer even for the fine remuneration it brings. Physicians carry the responsibility for life and death decisions. Thus, they must have complete confidence in their own knowledge and abilities in order to function with some sort of equanimity. Unfortunately, a few physicians transfer their complete confidence in their medical knowledge into areas where such confidence is not justified.

There is another small group of people who contribute to the confusion about toxicity of chemicals, but who are totally unrecognized by the general public. These are the scientists who devote their professional careers to analyzing (and often reinterpreting) toxicologic data produced by others, rather than engaging in productive research activities themselves. These scientists can provide a very valuable service to the public and their peers if their reviews are objective and complete. But they add to the problems of public mistrust when their efforts are devoted to reinterpreting (and often misinterpreting) work done by others without adding new or useful information.

In addition to miscellaneous scientists and physicians who render toxicologic opinions, recent years have seen the emergence of a new breed of toxicologist, the environmentalist–lawyer who knows the vocabulary but not the substance of toxicology. These lawyers, speaking as though they are experts in toxicology, become well-known to the public because they appear often on popular talk shows and in news media reports. They are given credence by the public because they are presented as experts by entertainment and news media.

Finally, there are the "high priests," scientists who have taken up a cause, usually the protection of the environment and of all God's lesser creatures against the machinations of devil man, which they consider requires the elimination of the use of synthetic chemicals. Their gospel includes stories of the damaging effects of synthetic chemicals, and they preach it with a religious zeal and passion. Their sermons seldom contain flagrant lies, but by carefully selecting data that support their theses they present half-truths as truths.

Many instances of disagreement regarding the toxicity of chemicals and the hazards they pose would cease to exist if the judgments and opinions of those who claim toxicologic expertise, in the absence of knowledge of toxicologic principles, were excluded from the controversy. A major problem is that the public has no way of distinguishing between self-proclaimed and legitimate experts. Attempts by anyone, no matter how objective, to indicate who is expert and who is not, would only cause further controversy and worsen the problem. The public must ultimately rely on its own good judgment in deciding which experts to heed.

SCIENTISTS AS HUMAN BEINGS

Another reason for disagreement among scientists concerning the toxicity or carcinogenicity of chemicals is related to the fact that scientists are, after all, human beings. They are subject to the same misjudgments, incompetencies, and assorted frailties as all other human beings. Further, being human, they are capable of interjecting their failings into their science.

Science is generally viewed by the public as being some impersonal, independent, and immutable set of truths about the nature of all things. In actual fact, science is nothing more than a product of human inquiry. Science is the body of systematized knowledge obtained by study, observation, and experimentation, for the purpose of determining the laws and principles that govern the physical world and all of its component parts, animate and inanimate. In a science such as toxicology, in which absolute answers to many important questions cannot be answered with the tools and methods available, the judgments of scientists become all important. Two scientists can review the same data and interpret them differently, particularly if their educational backgrounds and professional experiences differ.

The reality that scientists, like engineers and electricians, carpenters and clerks, can be incompetent in their fields of endeavor is usually not recognized by the public. The fact is that a fair amount of bad science does find its way into print in scientific journals. Bad toxicologic science appears to have no bias. It seems to underestimate or overestimate adverse effects of chemicals to an equal degree. The public should recognize that in toxicologic literature as in all other written works the existence of a statement in print does not guarantee its accuracy.

Unfortunately, because scientists are human, they can also be corrupted. News reports of brilliant graduate students whose research findings promised some great scientific advance but were discovered to be based on falsified data, or of large, important toxicologic testing facilities that furnished toxicity data for studies never performed, certainly must diminish public confidence in science. Such episodes are not common, but they do exist. They demonstrate that it is apparently difficult for some scientists to remain objective in their science, particularly if they have a preconceived idea of what their experimental results should be, or what they would want them to be, or what the agency paying for the research would want them to be. The tragedy of such corruption is that it provides grist for the mills of those who profit from public distrust of synthetic chemicals.

THE ROLE OF BIAS

Scientists, like all human beings, can have widely differing political and social value systems. Some scientists find it difficult to separate their political and social attitudes, which they hold with great sincerity and conviction, from their science. Science is objective, but scientists are not necessarily so.

The vehemence with which an otherwise rational scientist can hold and blatantly express a biased attitude was shockingly displayed many years ago at a meeting sponsored by the University of California to explore the subject of integrating chemical and biological pest-control methods in agricultural production. During his presentation, a noted population biologist stated that the petrochemical industry is at about the intellectual and moral level of the people who sell heroin to high school kids (reported December 7, 1977, A spirited attack on pesticide use, *San Francisco Chronicle,* p. 5). Such inflammatory statements may be very effective in gathering followers to a cause, but they are also very destructive to the process of solving some very critical problems whose solutions are essential for the public good.

Social scientists have studied the role of bias in professional decisions, and numerous philosophical essays have been written on the subject. Some claim that it is not possible for a scientist to divorce himself from his social values when making scientific judgments. Yet the objectivity of scientists in their respective fields of scientific endeavor is of crucial importance to societal and political decisions that will be of service and benefit to society rather than to some ideological movement.

Perhaps bias engendered by political and social values is most prone to influence attitudes that relate to subjects outside the area of a scientist's expertise. Hopefully, the majority of scientists can remain aloof from their personal biases when rendering judgments about the impact on society of scientific data from their own fields of endeavor. The question of whether a scientist can be objective may properly be classed as a trans-scientific one that falls into the second or third causes cited by Dr. Weinberg, above.

INFLUENCE OF FUNDING SOURCES

Another and important (but often ignored and unstated) reason for disagreement about the potential hazards presented by chemicals relates to the sources and supply of research monies. The federal government and other public agencies budget large sums of money for study of the effects of chemicals on environmental and public health. Funds from these sources are very limited in quantity and, therefore, there is a tremendous amount of competition for them. Obviously, the money is going to be granted for study in areas where the greatest problems exist. For example, a grant proposal to study the biochemistry of a chemical that does not appear to be toxic or carcinogenic would probably not compete successfully with a similar proposal for a chemical suspected of being a carcinogen, even though the former may have much more wide-ranging public health interest and significance. It is in the vested interest of scientists whose support comes largely or totally from grants to stress, if not exaggerate, the problems that their subject area poses for the environment or the public.

The other large source of research funds comes from the chemical and allied industries. These industries spend a great deal of money in developing the toxicity data required for chemicals that are regulated by governmental agencies. These monies are usually given to private toxicity testing laboratories or to universities because the chemical industry has become quite sensitized to claims that its own research is biased. It is not in industry's self-interest, primarily from the point of view of product liability, to understate or hide the hazards posed by their products. Neither is it in their self-interest to award grants or contracts to scientists who are openly antagonistic toward their industry.

The divergent sources of research support, combined with the tremendous competition for limited funds, cannot help but generate disagreements among scientists concerning the nature and degree of toxic hazard posed by chemicals.

WHAT TO DO?

Health and other governmental agencies that deal directly with the public should bring the public into the evaluation and decision-making processes relating to health and environmental matters. People who have a sense of control over their own destinies are more likely to work cooperatively to solve problems. They are more able to understand and appreciate the tremendous difficulties faced by science and by regulatory agencies in protecting environmental health.

The public also has a responsibility to educate itself by studying all aspects of issues. People should investigate the backgrounds and fields of expertise of people who attempt to sway them to a point of view. The view may be accepted or rejected. Whichever is the case, a person who has studied all sides of an issue can feel confident that the course he chooses is the proper one for him. An educated citizenry is the best insurance that decisions relating to environmental and public health protection will be of true and lasting benefit rather than just of immediate cosmetic value.

In conclusion, there are two rules for people who are interested in evaluating conflicting statements on adverse effects of chemicals: First, know the source. If a statement is made by someone noted for espousing a particular cause, regardless of whether it is prochemical or antichemical in nature, beware—his bias may be coloring his statements. Second, become informed. Learn all you can about the subject. There are many good books and other sources of information available to the public. An informed person is not at the mercy of propagandists and, as a result, is better able to make more effective and more competent decisions.

Appendix A

ABBREVIATIONS

AAF	acetyl amino fluorene
ACGIH	American Conference of Governmental Industrial Hygienists
ADI	acceptable daily intake
AHH	aryl hydrocarbon hydroxylase
ALD	average lethal dose
BAL	British Anti-Lewisite
CPSC	Consumer Product Safety Commission
2,4-D	2,4-dichloro phenoxy acetic acid
DD	dibenzodioxin
DDD	dichloro diphenyl dichloroethane
DDE	dichloro diphenyl dichloroethylene
DDT	dichloro diphenyl trichloroethane
DF	dibenzofuran
DMSO	dimethyl sulfoxide
DNA	deoxyribo nucleic acid
DOL	Department of Labor
DOT	Department of Transportation
EDF	Environmental Defense Fund
EDTA	ethylene diamine tetra acetate
EPA	Environmental Protection Agency
F	Fahrenheit
FDA	Food and Drug Administration
FDCA	Food, Drug, and Cosmetic Act
FIFRA	Federal Insecticide, Fungicide, and Rodenticide Act

ft^2	square foot
g	gram (about 0.035 ounces)
g/kg	grams of chemical per kilogram of feed or body weight
GRAS	generally regarded as safe
HSLA	Hazardous Substances Labeling Act
IU	international units
kg	kilogram (2.2 pounds)
l	liter (about 1 quart)
LC_{50}	lethal concentration for 50 percent of test animals
LD_{50}	lethal dose for 50 percent of test animals
lb	pound
m^2	square meter
m^3	cubic meter
MAC	maximum allowable concentration
mg	milligram (1/1,000th of a g)
mg/kg	milligrams per kilogram (of feed or body weight)
mg/l	milligrams per liter
mg/m^2	milligrams per square meter
mg/m^3	milligrams per cubic meter
μg	microgram (1/1,000th of a mg)
$\mu g/m^2$	micrograms per square meter
MLD	mean lethal dose
NCI	National Cancer Institute
NCTR	National Center for Toxicological Research
ng	nanogram (1/1,000th of a μg)
NIH	National Institutes of Health
NIOSH	National Institute for Occupational Safety and Health
NRDC	Natural Resources Defense Council
OSHA	Occupational Safety and Health Administration
oz	ounce
PCB	polychlorinated biphenyl
PCC	Poison Control Center
ppb	parts per billion
ppm	parts per million
ppt	parts per trillion
RfD, RFD	reference dose
RNA	ribonucleic acid
2,4,5-T	2,4,5-trichlorophenoxy acetic acid
tbsp	tablespoon
TCA	tricarboxylic acid
TCDD	tetrachloro dibenzodioxin

TCDF	tetrachloro dibenzofuran
TD_1	tumor dose for 1 in 100 individuals
TD_{50}	tumor dose for 50 in 100 individuals
TLV	threshold limit value
TOCP	tri-*ortho*-cresyl phosphate
tsp	teaspoon
USDA	U.S. Department of Agriculture
WHO	World Health Organization

Appendix B

TABLE OF EQUIVALENTS

kg	=	1,000 g, 1 million mg, 2.2 lbs
g	=	1,000 mg, 1 million μg, approx. 0.035 oz
mg	=	1,000 μg, 1 million ng
μg	=	1,000 ng

l	=	approx. 1 quart, approx. 33 oz
lb	=	16 oz, 454.5 g, 0.45 kg
oz	=	28.4 g

When referring to the concentration of a chemical in food or other medium:

mg/kg	=	ppm, μg/g
mg/l	=	ppm
μg/kg	=	ppb, ng/g
ng/kg	=	ppt
ppm	=	mg/kg, μg/g
ppb	=	μg/kg, ng/g
ppt	=	ng/kg

Appendix C

HOW MANY MOLECULES?

In order to understand how to calculate the number of molecules in any quantity of a chemical, two terms must be defined. One term is mole and the other term is Avogadro's number. A mole of any compound is its molecular weight expressed in grams. The molecular weight of a compound is the sum of the weights of its component atoms. For example, a water molecule is composed of two atoms of hydrogen (atomic weight of hydrogen is 1) and one atom of oxygen (atomic weight of oxygen is 16); thus, the molecular weight of water is 18 and a mole of water weighs 18 grams (a little over .5 ounce). A molecule of table salt is made up of one atom of sodium (atomic weight of sodium is 22) and one atom of chlorine (atomic weight of chlorine is 35); thus, a mole of salt weighs 57 grams, or a little less than 2 ounces.

Avogadro's number is a very confusing concept, even to chemistry students, because it is so very large: 6×10^{23} (6 with 23 zeros after it). But if one just thinks of Avogadro's number as a term that only refers to a specific number, like *dozen* or *gross,* it becomes easier to deal with. A dozen means 12, a gross means 144, and Avogadro's number means 6×10^{23}.

The number of molecules in a mole of any compound is equal to Avogadro's number. The weight of a mole will vary depending on the compound, just as the weight of a dozen will vary depending on what the dozen consists of, but the number of molecules in a mole is always the same. A dozen automobiles weighs tremendously more than a dozen eggs, but there are the same number of each. Thus, there are 6×10^{23} molecules of water in 18 grams of water and 6×10^{23} molecules of salt in 57 grams of table salt even though the weight of a mole of water is only about a third of the weight of a mole of salt.

A charcoal-broiled steak contains about 10 μg of benzpyrene. The number of molecules in 10 μg benzpyrene is calculated as follows: The molecular weight of benzpyrene is 252; therefore, a mole would weigh 252 grams; 252 g is equal to 2.52×10^8 μg (2.52000000 μg). The number of molecules in 1 μg is obtained by dividing the number of molecules in a mole by the number of μg in a mole. For benzpyrene, 6×10^{23} molecules in a mole divided by 2.52×10^8 μg in a mole equals 2.4×10^{15} molecules in a μg. The number of molecules in 10 μg benzpyrene would be 10 times as much, or 2.4×10^{16}.

Appendix D

FEDERAL AGENCIES AND THE SUBSTANCES THEY REGULATE

Agency	*Categories of Substances*
Consumer Product Safety Commission (CPC)	Flammable fabrics; children's products; all consumer products regulated by the Hazardous Substances Labeling Act (any product not regulated by food, drug, cosmetic, pesticide, or other laws) that are packaged in containers of a size that could reasonably be brought into a home, and that fit the Act's definition of hazard. HSLA covers a wide variety of products, including soaps, detergents, cleansers, bleaches, polishes, paints, hobby products, automotive products, and solvents
Department of Agriculture (USDA)	All commercial meat and meat products; poultry; dairy products.
Department of Transportation (DOT)	All hazardous chemicals, as defined by DOT regulations, while they are in transit.
Environmental Protection Agency (EPA)	All pesticides; pesticide residues on raw agricultural products; drinking water standards; air, water, soil pollutants; hazardous waste cleanup and disposal; all toxic industrial substances.

Food and Drug Administration (FDA)	Food additives; all processed foods, both human and pet; drugs; biologicals; cosmetics; medical devices.
National Institute for Occupational Safety and Health (NIOSH)	Investigates hazards in the workplace and makes recommendations for occupational safety and health standards.
Occupational Safety and Health Administration (OSHA)	Regulates safety and labeling of chemicals in the workplace; promulgates occupational safety and health standards and enforces these in the workplace.
American Conference of Governmental Industrial Hygienists (ACGIH)	Although ACGIH is not a federal agency, it is included here because of its impact on federal regulations dealing with chemicals in the workplace. ACGIH is a nonprofit, professional association which, for over five decades, has performed an extremely valuable public service by providing industrial hygienists with scientific information on effects of occupational exposure to chemical and physical agents. ACGIH publishes a booklet of threshold limit values (TLVs) that is updated yearly to include the latest scientific information on chronic toxicity and carcinogenicity of chemicals. TLVs are used to determine safe exposures to occupational chemicals. TLVs are not intended by ACGIH as legal standards, but, because of the prestige of ACGIH, most or all TLVs are accepted by both labor and industry and by regulatory agencies.

GLOSSARY

abortifacient: an agent that produces an abortion

abortus: the aborted products of conception.

abscissa: the horizontal axis (line) on a graph.

aerosol: a suspension of very small particles of a liquid or a solid in a gas.

adrenal glands: a pair of glands, sitting one on top of each kidney, that produce steroids, hormones related to metabolic functions, and adrenaline.

alchemy: a primitive medieval science remembered primarily for its search for a method for converting base metals into gold.

alveolus, alveoli (pl.): microscopic air sacs that form the terminal ends of the air passages of the lungs.

amalgam: an alloy of mercury with another metal, the most commonly known of which is the silver amalgam used for dental fillings.

ambient: surrounding. When applied to air, it means outdoor air.

amino acid: organic compounds that contain an acid grouping and an amine grouping. Amino acids are the building blocks of proteins.

analogous: similar or resembling each other in some way.

anaphylatic: pertaining to an extreme allergic reaction.

anatomic: pertaining to the structure of an organism.

angina pectoris: literally, pain in the chest; usually taken to mean heart pains.

anomaly: a thing or organism that deviates from normal.

antagonism: an interaction between two chemicals that results in one lessening the toxic effect of the other.

anthropomorphic: attributing human characteristics or form to nonhuman things.

anticoagulant: a chemical that prevents clotting of the blood.

aqueous: watery, or pertaining to a water solution.

aromatic: in organic chemistry, compounds that contain one or more benzene rings.

aspirate: to inhale liquid into the lungs.

atom: the smallest unit of an element that still maintains the physical and chemical properties of the element.

atrophy: to decrease in size or waste away.

avian: pertaining to birds.

benign: harmless.

bile: a liquid secreted by the liver.

bile duct: the tube that carries bile from the liver to the small intestine.

biochemical: a chemical produced by a living process.

biodegradable: capable of being metabolized by a biologic process or organism.

biodegradation: the process whereby chemicals are broken down by a biologic process or organism.

brominated: pertaining to the presence of one or more atoms of the element, bromine, in a compound.

caffeine: a naturally occurring stimulant found in coffee, tea, and cola nuts.

carcinogenic: capable of causing cancer.

cardiovascular: pertaining to the heart and blood vessels.

castration: removal of the testes or ovaries.

chloracne: a skin disease, resembling the acne of adolescence, caused by exposure to chlorinated aromatic organic compounds.

chlorinated: pertaining to the presence of one or more atoms of the element chlorine in a compound.

chromosome: one of the group of structures that form in the nucleus of a cell during cell division. Chromosomes, composed of DNA, carry the genetic code for the organism.

-cide: a suffix meaning "killer."

cilium, cilia: microscopic hairlike cellular projections that are capable of sweeping movement.

colic: acute abdominal pain.

colitis: inflammation of the large intestine (colon).

compound: a chemical substance composed of molecules all of the same kind.

confidence level: a statistical term that expresses how assured one can be that results obtained from an experiment did not occur by chance. For example, a 95 percent confidence level says that there is a 95 percent probability that the results obtained were due to the conditions of the experiment, and a 5 percent probability that they were due to chance.

congenital: pertaining to a condition existing before or at birth.

coumarin: a naturally occurring anticoagulant compound.

cytoplasm: cellular material within the cell membrane and surrounding the nucleus.

dam: the term used when referring to a laboratory animal mother.

DDD: dichloro diphenyl dichloroethane, a metabolite of DDT and itself a pesticide.

DDE: dichloro diphenyl dichloroethylene, a metabolite of DDT.

DDT: dichloro diphenyl trichloroethane, a chlorinated hydrocarbon pesticide, no longer permitted for general use in the United States.

demyelinate: to destroy or remove the sheath of fatlike material (myelin) that surrounds certain types of nerve fibers.

dermatitis: a skin inflammation.

dichotomy: a division into two mutually exclusive groups.

dielectric: pertaining to the nonconductance of electricity.

differentiation: in biology, the process whereby cells develop individual characteristics and become specialized in form or function, that is, liver cells, kidney cells, muscle cells.

DNA: the biochemical molecules (deoxyribo nucleic acids) from which chromosomes are made. Chromosomes, located in cell nuclei, carry the genetic code.

dosage: the regulation of doses, that is, how often, for how long.

dose: the quantity of chemical administered at one time.

dose–response curve: a graphic representation of the relationship between the dose administered and the effect produced.

dust: very small solid particles generated by grinding, crushing, or other mechanical processes.

edema: swelling due to collection of fluid in tissues.

electroencephalographic: pertaining to the diagnostic procedure in which a recording is made of brain waves.

electron: a subatomic particle that carries a negative charge.

element: a chemical substance composed of atoms of all the same kind.

embryo: an organism in the early stages of its development. In the human, it is the developing individual from conception to the end of the second month of uterine life.

emetic: an agent that induces vomiting.

empirical: based on experience and observation.

endemic: pertaining to prevalence in a particular region. An endemic disease is one that is constantly present at a low incidence in a particular region.

enzyme: a biochemical, usually protein, that speeds up the rate of biochemical reaction.

epidemiology: originally, the science that studied the cause and control of epidemics, outbreaks of a communicable disease in a region. Now, its subject matter includes diseases caused by chemicals and other environmental factors.

epigenetic (as used in this book): pertaining to a nongenetic mechanism.

epistemological: relating to the study of the methods and validity of knowledge.

esophagus: the tube that connects the mouth with the stomach.

estrogens: a group of female hormones.

ethanol: a naturally occurring 2-carbon alcohol, usually obtained from a fermentation process, and commonly known as alcohol.

etiology: the study of the causation of any disease.

extrapolation: the process of estimating unknown values from known values.

extrauterine: outside of the uterus.

feral: undomesticated; living in a wild state.

fetotoxic: toxic to a fetus.

fetus: the later stages of a developing organism. In the human, it is the unborn child during the period of uterine life from the end of the second month until birth.

fume: very small solid particles generated by recondensation of a vaporized solid.

fungicide: an agent that kills fungi, for example, molds, mildews, and mushrooms.

gas: individual molecules or atoms of a substance that has a boiling point below normal room temperature.

gastric: pertaining to the stomach.

gastrointestinal: pertaining to the stomach and intestines.

gene: the smallest subunit of a chromosome that contains a genetic message.

genome: the complete set of hereditary factors of an individual.

genotoxic: damaging to genetic material.

germicide: an agent that kills germs (pathogenic microorganisms).

germinal: pertaining to the reproductive cells.

gestation: pregnancy.

gonad: an organ that produces reproductive cells.

half-life: the length of time required for the quantity of the matter or property in question to be reduced by half.

hemoglobin: the red-colored biochemical in red cells that transports oxygen from the lungs to the tissues.

hemolysis: the rupture of red blood cell membranes that permits their contents to escape into the surrounding fluid.

hepatic portal vein: the blood vessel that carries blood from the intestinal walls to the liver.

hepatocarcinoma: cancer of the liver.

herbicide: an agent that kills plant life.

histopathology: the study of microscopic abnormalities produced by diseases.

homeostasis: the drive toward a steady state or equilibrium in the body.

homologus: similar or corresponding in some manner.

hormone: a biochemical secreted by one tissue in the body that exerts an influence on a biochemical function or organ somewhere else in the body.

hydroxylate: to introduce an oxygen–hydrogen group (hydroxyl group) into a molecule.

hyperkinesis: excessive activity or motion.

hyperpigmentation: the condition of having excess color in tissues or organs, such as the skin.

hypertrophy: excessive enlargement or overgrowth of an organ or tissue.

hypervitaminosis: an abnormal condition due to the excessive intake of one or more vitamins.

insecticide: an agent that kills insects.

isomer: a molecule that has the same number and kind of atoms as another molecule, but has a different arrangement of the atoms.

isotopes: atoms of the same element that differ in weight.

in utero: in the uterus (womb).

in vitro: in glass (test tube) or otherwise outside of a living organism.

in vivo: in a living organism.

lipids: organic chemicals that possess certain properties, such as being insoluble in water, commonly known as fats.

lipid-soluble: capable of being dissolved in fat or in solvents that dissolve fat.

lymphatic system: a system of vessels that originate in the tissues, drain the tissues of their clear fluids (lymph), and return the fluids back to the bloodstream at a site near the heart.

macromolecule: an extremely large molecule.

malaise: a vague feeling of discomfort or debility.

malignant: very injurious or deadly.

manometer: an instrument for measuring pressure.

megamouse: literally, a million mice; figuratively, a very large experiment.

menopause: literally, the cessation of menstrual periods. Menopause signals the end of a female's fertile life. In the human this period is also referred to as the change of life.

metabolism: the sum total of the biochemical reactions that a chemical undergoes in an organism.

metabolize: to undergo biochemical change in an organism.

metastasis: the spread of a disease to another part of the body.

methemoglobin: an oxidized form of hemoglobin that is not capable of transporting oxygen.

millirem: a thousandth of a rem (roentgen equivalent man), a unit of ionizing radiation which, when delivered to humans, is biologically equivalent to one thousandth of a roentgen of X- or gamma radiation (see roentgen).

mist: very small liquid droplets suspended in air.

mole: the molecular weight of a compound expressed in grams.

molecular weight: the weight of a molecule, calculated by adding the individual weights of all of the component atoms.

molecule: the smallest unit of a compound that still retains the physical and chemical properties of the compound.

monosaccharide: the simplest molecules of sugars, the building blocks of complex sugars such as starch and glycogen.

morbidity: the relative incidence of a disease in a population.

mortality: the relative incidence of deaths in a population.

mutagenic: pertaining to the ability to produce change, particularly genetic change.

mutant: an organism that has undergone a genetic change.

narcosis: the state of stupor or unconsciousness produced by a chemical.

nasopharynx: the area in back of the nose and above the opening of the mouth into the throat.

nausea: stomach upset accompanied by a feeling that one is about to vomit.

neoplasm: literally, a new growth. A neoplasm, also called a tumor, results from a more rapid than normal division of one or a few cells. A neoplasm may be benign or malignant.

no-effect level: as used in this book, a quantity of chemical that is below the threshold on the dose–response curve.

nomenclature: a list of names and words used in a specialized field.

nontarget: any object not intended to be hit. When used in reference to pesticide applications, nontarget means any object or organism that is not intended to be sprayed with pesticide.

ocular: pertaining to the eye.

oncogene: a gene that participates in a cancer process.

origin: the point on a graph that represents zero on both the vertical and horizontal axes (lines).

osteoporosis: a condition in which bones become less dense, and hence more fragile.

oxalic acid: a naturally occurring organic acid.

ozone: a gas composed of molecules of triatomic oxygen (O_3), the most reactive form of oxygen.

pandemic: epidemic disease spread over many regions.

paranoia: a mental disorder characterized by delusions.

parasympathetic: pertaining to part of the nervous system, below the level of consciousness, that participates in the regulation of the involuntary functions of the body, for example, heartbeat, breathing rate.

pathologic: pertaining to a disease state.

pentose sugar: a monosaccharide containing 5 carbon atoms in its structure.

peripheral nerves: the nerves that occur in the outer parts of the body, as opposed to those that occur in the brain and spinal column.

peritoneal cavity: the abdominal cavity that contains such organs as stomach, intestines, and liver.

pesticide: an agent used to kill pests. The category, pesticide, contains many -cides.

petrochemical: a chemical derived from petroleum.

pH: a term used to express the degree of acidity or alkalinity of a solution. A pH of 7 is neutral. Acid solutions have a pH below 7 and alkaline solutions have a pH greater than 7.

pharmaceutical: a therapeutic drug.

phylogenetic: pertaining to the evolutionary relationship among organisms.

physiologic: pertaining to the functions performed within living organisms.

placenta: the organ that forms the bridge between the fetal and the maternal bloodstreams.

pneumonitis: inflammation of the lungs.

poison: a chemical that is very highly toxic acutely. Legally, a chemical with an oral LD_{50} of 50 mg/kg or less.

polycyclic: in chemistry, pertaining to organic compounds whose molecules contain more than one circular structure (ring).

polymer: a large molecule (macromolecule) formed from the chemical combination of many smaller molecules, usually of only a few kinds. Proteins, starch, and cellulose are examples of natural polymers.

polyneuritis: inflammation of many nerves at the same time.

potable: suitable for drinking.

precursor: in biochemistry, a chemical from which another chemical is made.

primate: a member of the highest order of mammals, including man, apes, and monkeys.

prognosis: a forecast as to the probable outcome of an illness.

protocol: in science, the rules and outline of an experiment.

puberty: The period in which sexual maturity is attained.

purine: a family of complex organic chemicals composed of carbon, hydrogen, and nitrogen, arranged in two rings.

pyrimadine: like the purines, with the exception that the structure contains only one ring.

qualitative: pertaining to kind or type.

quantitative: pertaining to amount or degree.

quicksilver: the ancient name for the element, mercury.

radiomimetic: imitating ionizing radiations.

rectum: the portion of the large intestine (colon) just before it opens to the outside of the body (anus).

RNA: the biochemical molecules (ribonucleic acids) present in the cytoplasm of cells that function with DNA in carrying genetic information.

rodent: one of a group of gnawing mammals that includes rats, mice, rabbits, guinea pigs and hamsters.

rodenticide: an agent that kills rodents.

roentgen: a unit of X- or gamma radiation that describes the degree of ionization that results under certain specified conditions, named for the discoverer of X-rays, Wilhelm Roentgen (1845–1923).

respirable: capable of being inhaled.

sassolite: a mineral form of the element, boron.

scrotal: pertaining to the anatomic sac that holds the testes.

solanine: a naturally occurring chemical that occurs in potatoes and related species.

somatic: pertaining to body cells, as opposed to reproductive cells.

sublethal: pertaining to a dose level that is less than an amount necessary to cause death.

substrate: a chemical that serves as the substance acted upon by an enzyme.

synergism: an interaction between two chemicals that results in one enhancing the toxic effects of the other.

synthetic: made by humans.

systemic: pertaining to parts of an organism that unite in a common function.

teleologist: a person who believes that natural phenomena are directed to an end or shaped by a purpose.

teratogenic: pertaining to the ability to produce birth defects.

teratologist: a scientist who studies the causes of birth defects.

teratology: the study of abnormal embryological development and congenital malformations.

therapeutic: pertaining to the art of healing.

therapeutic index: the toxic dose of a drug divided by its curative dose. The greater the ratio, the safer the drug.

threshold: as used in this book, the point on a dose–response curve, above which effects occur and below which no effect occurs.

tolerance: the concentration of a pesticide residue or food additive permitted by regulations of EPA and FDA, respectively, to be in a specific food product.

uterine: pertaining to the uterus (womb).

vector: in biology, an object, organism, or thing that transmits disease from one host to another.

volatile: readily convertible to a vapor or gas form.

xenobiotic: foreign to life.

SUGGESTED READING

Barrons, Keith C. 1982. *Are Pesticides Really Necessary*. Chicago: Regnery Gateway.

Calabrese, Edward J. 1978. *Pollutants and High Risk Groups: The Biological Basis of Increased Human Susceptibility to Environmental and Occupational Pollutants*. New York: Wiley-Interscience.

Cancer Statistics: For information on books and pamphlets available on cancer risks and rates published by the NCI, NIH, and U.S. Department of Health and Human Services, contact your public library or the U.S. Government Printing Office, Washington, D.C. 20402.

Cohrssen, John J., and Vincent T. Covello. 1989. *Risk Analysis: A Guide to Principles and Methods for Analyzing Health and Environmental Risks*. Washington, D.C.: Council on Environmental Quality, Executive Office of the President.

Commoner, Barry. 1990. *Making Peace with the Planet*. New York: Pantheon.

Covello, V. T., and F. Allen. 1988. *Seven Cardinal Rules for Risk Communication*. Washington, D.C.: U.S. Environmental Protection Agency, Office of Policy Analysis.

Covello, V. T., D. von Winterfeldt, and P. Solvic. 1987. Communicating risk information to the public. In *Risk Communication: Proceedings of the National Conference on Risk Communication*. V. T. Covello, F. Allen, and J. C. Davies, eds. Washington, D.C.: The Conservation Foundation.

Douglas, Mary, and Aaron Wildavsky. 1982. *Risk and Culture*. Berkeley: University of California.

Efron, Edith. 1985. *The Apocalyptics*. New York: Touchstone/Simon & Schuster.

Epstein, Samuel S. 1979. *The Politics of Cancer*. Garden City, NY: Anchor/Doubleday.

Fraumeni, Joseph F., Jr., ed. 1975. *Persons at High Risk of Cancer*. New York: Academic Press.

Freudenthal, Ralph I., and Susan Loy Freudenthal. 1989. *What You Need to Know to Live with Chemicals.* Green Falls, CT: Hill and Garnett.

Heiby, Walter A. 1988. *The Reverse Effect.* Deerfield, IL: MediScience.

Hood, Ronald David, ed. 1990. *Developmental Toxicology.* New York: Van Nostrand Reinhold.

Hunter, Donald. 1975. *The Diseases of Occupations,* 5th ed. London: Hodder and Stoughton.

Jelliffe, E. F. P., and D. B. Jelliffe, eds. 1982. *Adverse Effects of Foods.* New York: Plenum.

Lowrance, William W. 1976. *Of Acceptable Risk: Science and the Determination of Safety.* Los Altos, CA: William Kaufamann.

Mizel, Steven B., and Peter Jaret. 1985. *In Self-Defense.* New York: Harcourt Brace Jovanovich.

Moore, Mike, ed. 1989. *Health Risks and the Press.* Washington, DC: The Media Institute.

Office of Technology Task Force. 1990. *Reproductive Hazards in the Workplace.* New York: Van Nostrand Reinhold.

Pachter, Henry M. 1951. *Magic into Science: The Story of Paracelsus.* New York: Henry Schuman.

Roueché, Berton. 1966. *Eleven Blue Men,* 13th print. New York: Berkley.

Schiefer, H. B., D. J. Irvine, and S. C. Buzik. 1987. *You and Toxicology.* Canada: University of Saskatchewan.

Slovic, P., B. Fischhoff, and S. Lichtenstein. 1980. Facts and fears: Understanding perceived risk. In *Social Risk Assessment: How Safe Is Safe Enough?* R. Schwing and W. A. Albers, eds. New York: Plenum Press.

Whelan, Elizabeth M. 1985. *Toxic Terror.* Ottawa, IL: Jamison.

Wildavsky, Aaron. 1988. *Searching for Safety.* New Brunswick, NJ: Transaction.

Williams, Roger J. 1967. *You Are Extraordinary.* New York: Random House.

Williams, Roger J. 1977. *Biochemical Individuality.* Austin, TX: University of Texas.

Williams, Roger J. 1977. *The Wonderful World Within You.* New York: Bantam.

Winter, C. K., J. N. Seiber, and C. F. Nuckton, eds. 1990. *Chemicals in the Human Food Chain.* New York: Van Nostrand Reinhold.

Wurtman, R. J., M. J. Baum, and J.T. Potts, eds. 1985. *The Medical and Biological Effects of Light.* New York: New York Academy of Sciences.

INDEX